Acupuncture: Visible Holi

Holism, the concept that Humanity, Society, and Nature form a unified system, each part embodying the whole and governed by the same laws, is central to both traditional Chinese medicine and the ancient Chinese philosophy from which it arose. Acupuncture, in its use of the laws of the macrocosm (Nature) to cure the ills of the microcosm (the human body), offers a tangible expression of this holistic world view. The practice of needling the lower part of the body to cure the upper, and treating the outer to heal the inner – cultivating the Root to nourish the Tip – is nothing less than holism made visible. Contemporary acupuncturists have inherited and continue to practice not only a unique and comprehensive system of medicine, but the entire Chinese holistic tradition upon which it is based.

Senior commissioning editor: Mary Seager
Development editor: Caroline Savage
Production controller: Anthony Read
Desk editor: Angela Davies
Cover design: Helen Brockway

Acupuncture: Visible Holism

an original interpretation of
acupuncture from Root to Tip

Bai Xinghua

with RB Baron

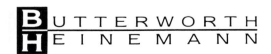

OXFORD   AUCKLAND   BOSTON   JOHANNESBURG   MELBOURNE   NEW DELHI

Butterworth-Heinemann
Linacre House, Jordan Hill, Oxford OX2 8DP
225 Wildwood Avenue, Woburn, MA 01801-2041
A division of Reed Educational and Professional Publishing Ltd

℞ A member of the Reed Elsevier plc group

First published 2001

British Library Cataloguing in Publication Data
A catalogue record for this book is available from the British Library

Library of Congress Cataloguing in Publication Data
A catalogue record for this book is available from the Library of Congress

ISBN 0 7506 4539 3

Composition by Genesis Typesetting, Laser Quay, Rochester, Kent
Printed and bound in Great Britain by Biddles Ltd, Guildford and King's Lynn

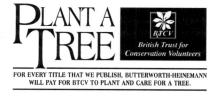

Contents

About the Authors

Bai Xinghua was born is a small village in Northeastern China in 1964. He completed his Bachelor's degree in Medicine in 1986 and his Master's degree in Acupuncture (at the Beijing University of Traditional Chinese Medicine) in 1989. He has been working as a lecturer and acupuncturist since 1989. He is a member of the Chinese Association of Acupuncture and Moxibustion, and has published numerous articles and books on the subject of traditional Chinese medicine (TCM). His works in English include *Chinese Auricular Therapy* (Scientific and Technical Documents Publishing House, Beijing, 1994) and *Acupuncture in Clinical Practice* (Butterworth-Heinemann, Oxford, 1996).

RB Baron, of Albion, California, USA, received her Bachelor's degree in Modern Chinese History from the University of California-Santa Cruz in 1991. She has been dividing her time between China and the United States since 1991, and has translated a wide range of Chinese literary and scientific materials into English. She collaborated with Dr Bai on both *Chinese Auricular Therapy* and *Acupuncture in Clinical Practice*.

Acknowledgements

I wish to express my heartfelt thanks to the following people, whose assistance was essential in making this book a reality.

My English language consultant and writing partner, RB Baron of Albion (California, USA) provided unfailing support and encouragement. She not only revised and edited the entire manuscript, but also clarified some original ideas so that Western readers can accept them with ease.

Mr Karl Juhnke gave very valuable suggestions on the general organization of the book, and edited the fourth chapter.

Ira Martin (Virginia, USA) sent me extensive English material concerning the history of world medicine, particularly the Hippocratic tradition. Readers will find these valuable references throughout the book, especially in the first chapter.

Ms Zi Mingjie generously shared her time with me to discuss and clarify some original ideas in the book.

Elisabeth Frei and Christine Reist provided me with both financial and moral support in times of difficulty.

Alan Baron provided material and feedback on acupuncture from the empiricists' camp, and he and Rose Marie Baron provided crucial financial assistance.

Mary Seager, Caroline Savage and Angela Davies of Butterworth-Heinemann (Oxford, UK) provided very professional support and advice.

Ms Jia Jie drew excellent illustrations.

Dr Wang Qianjin of the Natural Sciences History Institute of the Chinese Academy of Sciences clarified some longstanding questions concerning the geographical map.

Mr Chen Chengyong of the China Cartographic Publishing House helped computerize the ancient geographical map and the timeline.

The famous calligrapher Mr Li Zheng drew the Chinese characters that appear on the front cover: ... *Zhendao Ziran* – 'The Tao of Needling is modeled after Nature'.

RB Baron thanks Zattu, without whom she wouldn't have lived to tell the tale; Shadoh for holding down the fort; and Da Ming for bringing love, beauty, and rock and roll to her life.

She also gives her deepest thanks to her parents, Rose Marie and Alan Baron of Milwaukee (Wisconsin, USA) for their unconditional love, support and good humor through the years.

Finally, I want to thank my wife Cheng Guili, who gives me loving support and dedication.

Introduction

Healing therapies often resemble popular songs. They burst onto the scene and are heard on everyone's lips, only to fade just as quickly into obscurity. Acupuncture, on the other hand, is like a classical symphony. It has been practiced since its inception in China over 2000 years ago, and will continue to thrive all over the world throughout the new millennium.

Acupuncture has inspired a vast body of literature concerning both its theory and practice. It is quite difficult to discover anything new about the discipline. Nevertheless, this book will offer a groundbreaking new theory concerning the origins of acupuncture, as well as unique expositions of a number of important questions and an introduction of the entirely new concept of acupuncture as 'visible holism'.

Most people, when they encounter acupuncture, are primarily interested in what conditions it can treat and how it works. Few pause to wonder about its origins – when, and more importantly, *why* the ancient Chinese began to treat diseases by puncturing the body with bare needles. Even scholars have paid little attention to these questions; most textbooks on acupuncture and traditional Chinese medicine (TCM) mention them only in passing.

According to standard theory, acupuncture had its origins early in the Late Stone Age (the Neolithic Age, *c*. 8000–3500 BC) and developed gradually over many thousands of years through a process of trial and error. The traumatic nature of acupuncture, which may appear quite crude by modern standards, as well as its long history in China, seem to lend credence to these assumptions. However, if the accepted knowledge is correct, we are confronted with a great mystery. Why did acupuncture, unlike any other healing system, appear only in ancient China and nowhere else in the classical world?

This mystery was the seed of my research, and the book you now hold is the fruit of my investigations. Following a thorough study of the historical background of acupuncture, including ancient documents and recent archeological finds, I have become convinced that the standard theory concerning its origins and development is untenable. I believe that acupuncture is by no means a purely empirical healing method that evolved gradually during prehistoric times. On the contrary, it was a great and relatively sudden invention based on theory as well as practice, which occurred in classical China during the early Western Han Dynasty (206 BC–24 AD), not long before the birth of Christ.

The Western Han Dynasty arose over 2000 years ago. This is a considerable span of time in the overall history of human civilization. However, in the context of China's 4000 years of recorded history, the civilization of the Western Han was actually more modern than primitive. The previous centuries had seen the blossoming of Chinese culture during the intellectual give-and-take of the Spring and Autumn (770–476 BC) and Warring States

(475–221 BC) Periods, and the subsequent territorial unification of China by the Qin Dynasty (221–207 BC) laid a foundation for the cultural integration of the diverse states. Acupuncture was one of the fruits of this rich period of Chinese history.

Many aspects of Chinese culture, including technology, geography, philosophy and social relations, contributed to the invention and development of acupuncture. For example, through their work with flood control the Chinese ancestors learned to use dredging to remove obstacles and direct the flow of water through riverbeds, the channels of the Earth. This led to the realization that needling could be similarly used to remove obstructions and stimulate the flow of *qi* through the meridians, the channels of the body. The holistic application of the same principle allowed the classical Chinese both to control flooding and to treat disease and disorder.

This intuitive association between the channels of the Earth (the macrocosm) and the channels of the body (the microcosm) may seem strange to modern readers, but holism, the awareness that each part mirrors the whole, was one of the most fundamental principles of classical Chinese philosophy. Chinese holistic thought regards humanity, society and Nature as an organic, unified whole. The human body is seen as a microcosmic image of Nature. It is believed that Human and Nature are similarly constituted and governed by the same laws, and that their disorders can therefore be similarly managed. The invention of acupuncture was a direct outgrowth of this holistic philosophy.

Acupuncture treats disease and disorder by needling specific acupoints along the meridians in order to stimulate the flow of *qi*, or life force, through these channels. Accepted theory holds that the development of acupuncture and the acupoints preceded the identification of the meridians. It is generally believed that fortuitous accidental injury and repeated empirical testing during the Neolithic Age (*c.* 8000–3500 BC) gradually revealed acupoints that were effective for treating various conditions. The meridians are thought to have been visualized much later as a hypothetical system linking previously discovered acupoints – connecting the dots, as it were.

However, recent archeological findings challenge this theory. Evidence indicates that the identification of the meridians actually predated the appearance of acupuncture, and was a crucial precondition for its invention and the discovery of the various acupoints.

The earliest known text on acupuncture and acupoints is The *Yellow Emperor's Inner Classic of Medicine* (*c.* 104–32 BC) (*Huang Di Neijing*, hereafter referred to as the *Neijing*), compiled during the Western Han Dynasty (206 BC–24 AD). No mention of either acupuncture or acupoints has been found in any prior medical documents. The first discussion of the meridians, however, occurs in a collection of much earlier texts, The *Ancient Medical Relics of Mawangdui* (*c.* prior to 168 BC). Furthermore, these texts refer only to the use of moxibustion, the application of heat, along the general pathways of the meridians to stimulate the flow of *qi*. They make no mention of either acupuncture or specific acupoints. This suggests that the ancient Chinese were familiar with moxibustion and the meridians well before they started to use acupuncture. Extensive further evidence, both classical and modern, exists to support this new hypothesis, and will be discussed in detail in this book.

Moxibustion, like acupuncture, treats disease and disorder by stimulating the flow of *qi* through the meridians. The two healing methods are so closely related that they are referred to by a single compound word in Chinese. However, the application of heat for healing is much more ancient than the use of needling. It seems quite reasonable to assume that moxibustion had its origins soon after the mastery of fire by Early Stone Age humans approximately 500 000 years ago (during the Paleolithic Age, *c.* 2 000 000–8000 BC), since it was at this time that humans were first able instinctively to apply warmth to relieve the pain of injury or disease.

My research has led me to believe that the identification of the meridians arose directly from the practice of moxibustion. It was through the application of moxibustion that the ancient Chinese first became aware of the phenomenon of meridian transmission, the sensation that occurs when the flow of *qi* is stimulated. Although this phenomenon, referred to in the *Neijing* as *deqi* (obtaining *qi*), is now popularly known as the 'needling sensation', it was actually first stimulated by heat rather than needles. The earliest descriptions of the pathways of the meridians recorded in the ancient medical documents are maps of these transmissions of *qi* through the body, stimulated by the application of heat.

Compared to moxibustion, acupuncture is quite traumatic and counterintuitive. The Chinese ancestors could not have made this revolutionary medical innovation prior to the breakthrough in understanding of the human body and Nature that occurred around the time of the Western Han Dynasty (206 BC–24 AD). Furthermore, it would not have been necessary for them to discover the acupoints before the advent of acupuncture, since moxibustion can easily be applied to a large area or along the entire course of a meridian. Acupuncture, however, requires the identification of discrete points through which the needles can be inserted. Acupoints were therefore the final aspect of acupuncture to be developed, well after moxibustion and the identification of the meridians.

Our reconsideration of the origins of acupuncture thus reveals a chronological progression leading from the first prehistoric applications of moxibustion to the identification of the meridians, and on to the invention of acupuncture and the discovery of the various acupoints.

In most acupuncture textbooks, acupuncture is defined as the use of needles to penetrate and stimulate specific points on the body in order to restore normal function and energetic balance. This concept is very superficial, expressing merely the form of acupuncture and not its essence. In this book, I will develop the completely new concept of acupuncture as 'visible holism'.

Holism is the core of ancient Chinese philosophy, and the theoretical basis of traditional Chinese medicine (TCM). It is an abstract concept that is invisible and difficult to understand. The practice of acupuncture offers a tangible expression of this intangible idea. The insertion of needles into discrete points of the body in order to effect a distal or systemic cure embodies the holistic relationship between the microcosm and macrocosm, as well as between the upper and lower parts and interior and exterior tissues of the body. Acupuncture in practice is holistic sculpture; it makes holism visible and concrete. It is not merely a healing art, but the expression of thousands of years of Chinese culture. Acupuncturists have the honor of inheriting and practicing not only a system of healing, but also the philosophy of holism.

As we enter the twenty-first century, our globe is rapidly becoming a small village. The cultures of various nations are becoming integrated, just as happened in China over two millennia ago. Chinese people are enjoying Western yogurt, while Westerners are embracing Chinese needling. Yogurt can be sweet and needling bitter, but both are beneficial to the health. The spread of acupuncture will not only improve the health of people around the planet, but also open their doors to traditional Chinese holistic thinking.

Chapter 1

The origins of acupuncture – a unique synthesis of Chinese culture

'The Tao of Needling is modeled after Nature.'
Lingshu

Acupuncture, the most important system of treatment in traditional Chinese medicine (TCM), has a recorded history that reaches back more than 2000 years. However, strangely enough there are no definitive historical or archeological records of its origins. It is as if acupuncture appeared out of nowhere, like a phenomenon of Nature. Many questions exist concerning this unique healing method. When and how did it first appear, develop, and mature into a complete therapeutic system? What were the conditions that resulted in its development only in China, and nowhere else in the classical world? This chapter presents a new theory concerning the origins of acupuncture, based on a new approach to the archeological evidence and the author's unique analysis of China's ancient system of flood control, as well as an exposition of the groundbreaking concept of acupuncture as visible holism.

Unique characteristics of acupuncture

Acupuncture is often used in conjunction with moxibustion in traditional Chinese medicine (TCM). The two techniques are so closely related that they are referred to in Chinese with one compound word, *zhenjiu* – acupuncture (*zhen*, needle) plus moxibustion (*jiu*, to burn). A new English word containing these two meanings, acumoxa, has recently been coined. However, the intrinsic differences between acupuncture and moxibustion make it necessary to consider their origins separately.

Moxibustion is a type of traditional Chinese medicine that treats disease and disorder by stimulating the acupoints and meridians with heat. The invention of moxibustion was directly related to the discovery and use of fire by prehistoric humans approximately 500 000 years ago, during the Paleolithic Age (*c.* 2 000 000–8000 BC). All animals, people included, instinctively prefer warmth and dislike cold. Even plants exhibit phototaxic or thermotoaxic properties. The application of heat for healing is universal and has been part of numerous recorded medical traditions, including those of classical Greece and Rome. At some point in prehistory, our ancestors discovered that fire could be used not only to cook their food and warm their bodies, but also to relieve or even cure their ills.

Acupuncture, which treats disease and disorder by puncturing the acupoints with needles, differs from moxibustion in the following ways.

Acupuncture is inherently traumatic

Many methods of pain relief, including the application of heat, have developed from instinctive human reactions, and appear imminently logical:

> An individual hurts his leg and spontaneously without thinking he rubs it . . . Another individual suffers from lumbago, crawls to the fire and as soon as he feels the heat the pain becomes more tolerable . . . We can well imagine that early man suffering an acute pain in the stomach felt impelled to act, pressed his epigastrium with both hands, applied heat or cold, or drank water or some decoction until he felt relieved. Pain, in other words, released a series of instinctive reactions, some of which were more effective than others. With developing civilization men learned to differentiate between treatments, became aware of them, remembered them and passed them on. Sigerist, 1983[1]

On the contrary, puncturing the body with needles is by no means an instinctive reaction when sick or in pain. Most people do not like needles and would prefer to avoid them. Many plants and animals have taken advantage of this natural response, and evolved thorns or quills as weapons to protect themselves from attack. Needling will cause some degree of physical trauma, no matter how fine the needle or skillful the practitioner. A modern report shows that when a needle 0.2 mm in diameter (the size of modern acupuncture needles) is used to puncture a rabbit, four to twenty muscle fibers and ten to twenty nerve fibers are damaged[2]. The degree of trauma was much greater in antiquity, when needles were much larger. Even in the more recent past acupuncture needles as thick as 2 mm in diameter were still occasionally used; in the late 1960s, the folk practitioner in my home village commonly used needles of this size. In the early 1980s, when I was an undergraduate student, I personally observed him insert this type of needle with both hands to treat a case of epigastric pain.

What seems even more illogical is that acupuncture is often applied distally, rather than locally. It is clear that the direct application of warmth can relieve local discomfort. It is also clear why it may be necessary to cause further trauma to an injured area in certain situations, such as when surgery is required or a broken bone must be set. It is however by no means obvious why acupuncture often calls for needling points far distant from the location of the problem. One of the principles of acupuncture instructs: 'Needle the lower to cure the upper'[3]. For instance, a common acupuncture treatment requires needling LI4-Hegu, located on the hand, to relieve toothache. It would seem to the layperson that the healthy hand has nothing to do with the diseased head, so why should it be traumatized? But once the principles of the meridians are understood, it becomes clear that the body is an integrated system, and that the trauma of inserting needles in one area of the body can produce the holistic effect of relieving problems elsewhere.

Although acupuncture can sometimes be painful, it causes no serious or lasting injury when carried out correctly. Many people are willing to endure the minor pain of needling in order to relieve a major problem. Unfortunately acupuncture may seem frightening to some, especially in the West where it is often misunderstood and misrepresented. For instance, the entry for acupuncture in as respected a source as the *Encyclopedia Americana* contains a picture of a man's head punctured with over seventy needles[4], although a properly trained and experienced acupuncturist would never needle in such an exaggerated and excessive manner.

Acupuncture is of uniquely Chinese origin

Among all the systems of holistic healing invented in the classical world, acupuncture alone was unique to China. There are no corresponding or even similar healing systems in the early medical traditions of other cultures. The four great inventions of ancient China (paper, the printing press, gunpowder and the compass) were all eventually duplicated independently in other parts of the globe. Even if these inventions hadn't first been made in China, compact discs, laser printing, nuclear weapons and global positioning satellites would still have been developed from these fundamental breakthroughs. However, without the invention of acupuncture in ancient China there would be no needling therapy today. Acupuncturists today still adhere to the same doctrines and manipulate needles in the same ways as their counterparts in the days of the *Neijing*, or *Yellow Emperor's Inner Classic of the Medicine*, the earliest known treatise on acupuncture (*c*. 104–34 BC). Despite the introduction of painless and non-invasive methods such as acupressure or point stimulation using electricity or short waves, needling has remained the primary treatment method in acupuncture.

The origins of acupuncture: challenging the accepted theory

The uniqueness and stability of acupuncture are unparalleled in the history of science throughout the world. Although many ancient civilizations besides China developed methods for treating disease and maintaining health, these ancient medical traditions have either been lost or survive only as remnants in modern alternative medicine. For example, it is said of Greek medicine that 'Ironically, the man who today is called "the father of medicine" [Hippocrates] has little influence over modern medical thinking. He is more apt to be cited as an inspiration by practitioners of alternative medicine, many of whom regard his fundamental precepts as still valid'[5].

The question that now arises is, how was acupuncture invented? Standard theory assumes that acupuncture had its origins early in the Late Stone Age (the Neolithic Age, *c*. 8000–3500 BC), and developed gradually over many thousands of years through a process of trial and error and empirical experience. The following is a typical explanation of the genesis of acupuncture, taken from a popular textbook on traditional Chinese medicine[6]:

> Acupuncture and moxibustion . . . originated as early as China's clan period in the Late Stone Age. During the Early Stone Age [Paleolithic Age, *c*. 2 000 000–8000 BC], from remote prehistory to [approximately 8000 BC], stone knives and scrapers [were used] to incise abscesses, drain pus, and let blood for therapeutic purposes . . . During the Late Stone Age, improvements in stone working techniques allowed the development of *bian* stones as specialized medical instruments . . . With the introduction of iron working during the feudal period [*c*. 500 BC–25 AD], *bian* stones were replaced by metal medical needles.

Although this depiction seems plausible, it is not based on factual evidence. Furthermore, it does not address several important questions.

Does the invention of acupuncture date from the Neolithic Age (*c*. 8000–3500 BC)?

Prior to the 1970s, the earliest references to acupuncture were found in China's oldest known medical treatise, The *Yellow Emperor's Inner Classic of the Yellow Emperor* (*Huang Di Neijing*, hereafter referred to as the *Neijing*) (*c*. 104–34 BC). The *Neijing* consists of two parts: *Suwen* – the *Simple Questions*, and *Lingshu* – the *Spiritual Pivot*, also known as *The Classic of Acupuncture* (*Zhenjing*). Although authorship of the *Neijing* is attributed to the legendary Yellow Emperor, Huang Di (*c.* 2650 BC), most scholars consider that this master work, which contains excerpts from more than twenty pre-existing medical treatises, was actually compiled between 104 BC and 32 BC, during the latter part of the Western Han Dynasty (206 BC–24 AD)[7]. In part because of the comprehensive and highly developed nature of the medical system presented in the *Neijing*, scholars of acupuncture have assumed that needling therapy has an extremely long history, probably reaching back to prehistoric times. Furthermore, the original versions of the ancient texts used in the compilation of the *Neijing* have been lost, and with them the opportunity to further illuminate the question of when acupuncture actually first appeared.

However, startling new archeological finds were made in China in the early 1970s, revealing the true state of medicine prior to the *Neijing*. In late 1973, fourteen medical documents known as the *Ancient Medical Relics of Mawangdui* were excavated from Grave No. 3 at Mawangdui on the outskirts of Changsha, Hunan Province. Ten of these

---

Figure 1.1   Meridians of the Earth: the meridians of the body in macrocosm.

This map shows the correspondence between the rivers of ancient China and the distribution of the meridians, as described in Chapter 12 of the *Lingshu*, 'Regular Watercourses'. It is based on a geographic map entitled *Yuji Tu* (*Map of Yu's Traces*), which was engraved on stone in 1136 AD. The stone map, a representation of the watercourses of ancient China, is named after the legendary Great Yu to commemorate his unparalleled accomplishments in flood control. This map was considered the most outstanding cartograph in the world at the time it was engraved. It is divided into a grid of 5110 equal squares. Each square is approximately 1.2 cm to a side, and corresponds to an area of approximately 10 000 square *li*, or 2500 square kilometers, a scale of approximately 1:4 500 000. The drawing of the coastline and main watercourses is quite exact, even when compared with modern geographic maps drawn using the global positioning system (GPS).

The birthplaces of eminent ancient physicians and philosophers and sites of recent archeological finds related to traditional Chinese medicine, particularly acupuncture and moxibustion, are marked on the map as follows:

1. Nine metal acupuncture needles (*c.* 113 BC), Mancheng County, Hebei Province, excavated in 1968
2. Bian Que (Qin Yueren) (*c.* 407–310 BC), legendary inventor of acupuncture. His name means Wayfaring Magpie, a bird which symbolizes good fortune. Renqiu County, Hebei Province
3. Sunzi (*c.* contemporary of Confucius, 551–479 BC), famous philosopher and military strategist. Huimin County, Shandong Province
4. Cang Gong (Chunyu Yi) (*c.* 215–140 BC), earliest recorded Chinese medical practitioner. Zibo, Shandong Province
5. Kongzi (Confucius) (551–479 BC), philosopher and founder of Confucianism. Qufu County, Shandong Province
6. Mengzi (Mencius) (*c.* 385–304 BC), philosopher and follower of Confucius. Zhou County, Shandong Province
7. Xunzi (*c.* 298–238 BC), philosopher. Changshan County, Shandong Province
8. Huangfu Mi (*c.* 215–282 AD), acupuncturist and author of the *Systematic Classic of Acupuncture and Moxibustion*. Lingtai County, Gansu Province
9. Sima Qian (*c.* 135–???), eminent historian and author of the *Historical Records*. Hancheng County, Shanxi Province
10. Zhuangzi (*c.* 369–286 BC), philosopher and follower of Laozi. Shangqiu, Henan Province
11. Hua Tuo (*c.* 150–208 AD), famous surgeon and acupuncturist. Bo County, Anhui Province
12. Laozi (Lao Tzu) (*c.* sixth century BC), philosopher and founder of Taoism. Luyi County, Henan Province
13. Guanzi (*c.* 725–645 BC), earliest recorded Chinese philosopher. Yingshang County, Anhui Province
14. Zhang Ji (Zhang Zhongjing) (*c.* 150–219 AD), sage of Chinese medicine and author of *Discussion on Cold Induced Diseases*. Anyang, Henan Province
15. Lacquered wooden figure showing meridians (*c.* 100 BC). Mianyang, Sichuan Province, excavated in 1993
16. Guo Yu (*c.* 60–125 AD), early imperial acupuncturist. Guanghan County, Sichuan Province
17. *Book of the Meridians (Mai Shu)* (*c.* prior to 179 BC), written on bamboo slips. Jiangling County, Hubei Province, excavated in 1983
18. *Ancient Medical Relics of Mawangdui* (*c.* prior to 168 BC), written on silk and bamboo slips. Changsha, Hunan Province, excavated in 1973.

documents were hand-copied on silk, and four were written on bamboo slips. (See Appendices 1, 2 and 3.) These documents were probably lost some time during the Eastern Han Dynasty (25–220 AD), since no mention of them has been found in any medical documents from after this time.

The exact age of the *Ancient Medical Relics of Mawangdui* has not been determined. However, a wooden tablet found in the grave states that the deceased was the son of Prime Minister Li Chang of the state of Changsha, and that he was buried on 24 February, 168 BC. The unsystematic and empirical nature of the material contained in the *Relics* indicates that they were written well before they were buried in 168 BC, probably around the middle of the Warring States Period (475–221 BC)[8]. In any event, the *Relics* pre-date the *Neijing* (compiled *c*. 104–32 BC), making them the oldest medical documents in existence.

Another valuable medical find, *The Book of the Meridians* (*Mai Shu*), was excavated from two ancient tombs at Zhangjiashan in Jiangling County, Hubei Province in 1983.

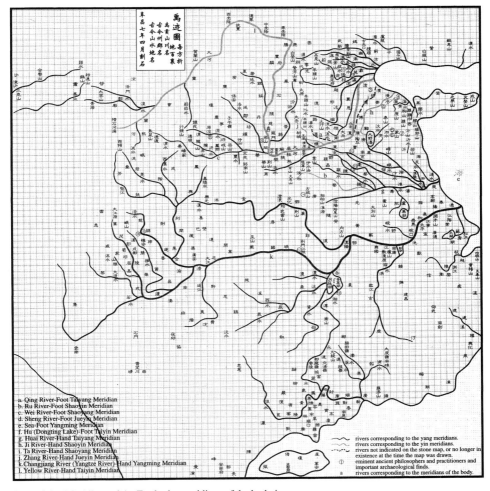

a. Qing River–Foot Taiyang Meridian
b. Ru River–Foot Shaoyin Meridian
c. Wei River–Foot Shaoyang Meridian
d. Sheng River–Foot Jueyin Meridian
e. Sea–Foot Yangming Meridian
f. Hu (Dongting Lake)–Foot Taiyin Meridian
g. Huai River–Hand Taiyang Meridian
h. Ji River–Hand Shaoyin Meridian
i. Ta River–Hand Shaoyang Meridian
j. Zhang River–Hand Jueyin Meridian
k. Changjiang River (Yangtze River)–Hand Yangming Meridian
l. Yellow River–Hand Taiyin Meridian

〜〜 rivers corresponding to the yang meridians.
〜〜 rivers corresponding to the yin meridians.
---〜 rivers not indicated on the stone map, or no longer in existence at the time the map was drawn.
① eminent ancient philosophers and practitioners and important archaeological finds.
     rivers corresponding to the meridians of the body.

Figure 1.1   Meridians of the Earth: the meridians of the body in macrocosm.

These ancient texts, written on bamboo slips and quite well preserved, were probably buried between 187 and 179 BC, approximately the same time as the Mawangdui relics[9]. There are five documents in all, three of which (*The Classic of Moxibustion with Eleven Yin-Yang Meridians*, *Methods of Pulse Examination and Bian Stone*, and *Indications of Death on the Yin-Yang Meridians*) are identical to texts from Mawangdui. (See Appendices 1, 2 and 3.)

China's first recorded medical practitioner, Cang Gong (*c.* 215–140 BC), came into possession of a number of these medical texts around 180 BC. (See Figure 1.1.) Cang Gong lived in Zibo, Shandong Province, over 1000 kilometers from both Mawangdui and Zhangjiashan. The fact that copies of these documents were present in such widely separated places around the same time provides further evidence that they were written and disseminated long before the date they were placed in the tombs.

There is abundant evidence to show that the authors of the *Neijing* used the *Ancient Medical Relics of Mawangdui* as primary references, further indicating the antiquity of the *Relics*. For example, Chapter 10 of the *Lingshu* section of the *Neijing* contains a discussion of the meridians and their disorders that is very similar, in both form and content, to that found in the *Classic of Moxibustion with Eleven Yin-Yang Meridians*, one of the documents of the *Ancient Medical Relics of Mawangdui*. (See Appendices 3 and 4.)

Of course, the *Neijing* did not simply reproduce these earlier documents, but rather refined and developed them, and introduced new therapeutic methods. The earlier *Classic of Moxibustion with Eleven Yin-Yang Meridians* is limited to moxibustion, while Chapter 10 of the *Lingshu* section of the *Neijing* mentions needling therapy, or acupuncture, for the first time. Although the therapies contained in the *Ancient Medical Relics of Mawangdui* are varied, including herbal medicine, moxibustion, fomentation, medicinal bathing, *bian* stone therapy, massage, *daoyin* (physical exercises), *xingqi* (breathing exercises), *zhuyou* (incantation)[10] and even surgery[11], there is no mention of acupuncture. This indicates that acupuncture was developed after moxibustion, and was probably not yet in existence at the time that the *Ancient Medical Relics of Mawangdui* were compiled.

If, as has generally been thought, needling therapy did indeed originate much earlier than the *Neijing* (*c.* 104–32 BC), references to acupuncture should also be found in earlier documents such as the *Ancient Medical Relics of Mawangdui* (*c.* prior to 168 BC). However, the *Relics* contain no such references, indicating that acupuncture was not yet in use at the time the *Relics* were compiled. Although it might be arbitrary to infer the actual condition of medicine early in the Western Han Dynasty (206 BC–24 AD) simply on the basis of the *Ancient Medical Relics of Mawangdui*, the fact that these documents were considered valuable enough to be buried with the deceased indicate that they do reflect general medical practices at the time.

The *Historical Records* (*Shi Ji*) (*c.* 104–91 BC) by Sima Qian contains evidence that acupuncture was first used approximately 100 years before the *Neijing* (*c.* 104–32 BC). It also contains biographies of the two earliest known Chinese medical practitioners, Bian Que and Cang Gong[12].

Bian Que's life was surrounded by an aura of mystery, which makes it difficult to separate fact from legend. His name means 'Wayfaring Magpie' – a bird that symbolizes good fortune. It is said that an old man gave Bian Que some secret medical books and an herbal prescription, and then disappeared. Bian Que took the medicine according to the mysterious visitor's instructions, and 30 days later he could see through walls. Thereafter when he diagnosed disease, he could clearly see the internal *zangfu* organs. Like the centaur Chiron (son of Apollo), who is sometimes regarded as the god of surgery in the West, Bian Que is considered to be a god of healing who is more than human. He is depicted with a human head and bird's body on a stone relief unearthed from a tomb of the Han Dynasty (206 BC–220 AD).

Bian Que's given name was Qin Yueren. It is known that he lived from 407–310 BC, during the late Warring States Period (475–221 BC), and was a contemporary of the father of the Western medicine, Hippocrates (*c.* 460–377 BC). The *Historical Records* states that Bian Que successfully resuscitated the prince of the State of Guo using a combination of acupuncture, fomentation and herbal medicine. Bian Que is thus considered to be the founder of acupuncture, making the first recorded use of acupuncture during the late Warring States Period (475–221 BC).

More solid evidence connects the birth of acupuncture with Chunyu Yi (*c.* 215–140 BC), popularly known as Cang Gong. His life and work are described in detail in the *Historical Records*. Sima Qian states that in 180 BC, Cang Gong's teacher gave him many precious medical books that had escaped the book-burnings of the last days of the Great Qin Empire (221–207 BC). At that time, adherents of all opposing schools of thought were executed or exiled, and almost all books not conforming to the rigid Legalist doctrines that dominated the dynasty were burned. Although medical books escaped the disaster, their owners were still afraid of persecution. The banned books that Cang Gong received might have included a number whose titles appear in the *Ancient Medical Relics of Mawangdui*, such as the *Classic of Moxibustion with Eleven Yin-Yang Meridians*, *Classic of Moxibustion with Eleven Foot-Arm Meridians*, *Method of Pulse Examination and Bian Stone*, *Therapeutic Methods for 52 Diseases*, *Miscellaneous Forbidden Methods*, and *The Book of Sex*.

Cang Gong's biography in the *Historical Records* discusses twenty-five of his cases, dating from approximately 186–154 BC. These medical cases, the earliest in recorded Chinese history, give a clear picture of how disease was treated over 2100 years ago. Of the twenty-five cases, ten were diagnosed as incurable and the patients died as predicted[13]. Of the fifteen that were cured, eleven were treated with herbal medicine, two with moxibustion in combination with herbal medicine, one with needling, and one with needling in combination with pouring cold water on the patient's head. It can be seen that Cang Gong used herbal medicine as his primary treatment, and acupuncture and moxibustion only secondarily.

Cang Gong's two moxibustion cases adhere strictly to the doctrines recorded in the *Ancient Medical Relics of Mawangdui* (*c.* prior to 168 BC). In the first case (a man with tooth decay), moxibustion was applied to the Hand Yangming Meridian to relieve pain, followed by gargling with a decoction of Flavescent Sophora to clean the mouth and kill worms. According to both the *Classic of Moxibustion with Eleven Yin-Yang Meridians* and the *Classic of Moxibustion with Eleven Foot-Arm Meridians* from the *Ancient Medical Relics of Mawangdui*, toothache is a primary disorder of the Hand Yangming Meridian, and moxibustion should be used on the affected meridian to relieve pain. (See Appendices 2 and 3.) The second case was a woman who suffered from difficult urination with yellow urine, accompanied by swelling and pain in the lower abdomen. Dr Cang diagnosed the condition as a disorder of the Foot Jueyin Meridian, and applied moxibustion on this meridian bilaterally. The pain was relieved immediately following the first treatment. This treatment is identical to that recorded in the *Classic of Moxibustion with Eleven Yin-Yang Meridians* from Mawangdui. (See Appendix 3.)

Although only two of Cang Gong's cases in which he employed moxibustion are recorded in the *Historical Records*, it is known that he was expert in its use, and that he wrote a book called *Cang Gong's Moxibustion*. Unfortunately, this book has been lost. The only surviving fragment is a treatment for epilepsy, preserved in *Essential Prescriptions Worth a Thousand Pieces of Gold*, written by Sun Simiao (*c.* 682 AD) during the Tang Dynasty (618–907 AD)[14].

In comparison with his wide-ranging utilization of herbal medicine and moxibustion, Cang Gong applied needling therapy very sparingly. One of two recorded cases in which Cang Gong used acupuncture was a king's mother who complained of hot feet and depression. Cang Gong diagnosed the condition as *rejue*, heat reversal, caused by overindulgence in alcohol. He therefore needled three areas on the sole of each foot, pressing the treated areas after withdrawal of the needles to avoid bleeding. All symptoms disappeared immediately after treatment. The other case was a man suffering from headache, fever and restlessness. After taking his pulse, Cang Gong ascertained that the condition was upward reversal of yang *qi*, which he believed was brought on by the patient going to bed with wet hair. He sprinkled cold water on the patient's head and needled three areas on the bilateral sides of the Foot Yangming Meridian in order to clear heat. The patient had a full recovery after one treatment.

Neither of Cang Gong's two recorded acupuncture cases mention specific acupoints or how the needles were manipulated, indicating that needling therapy at the time was still in its initial stage. However, both cases were cured with only one treatment, indicating the efficacy of the nascent therapy. The rapid development of acupuncture was soon to follow.

By the time the *Neijing* was compiled (*c.* 104–32 BC), approximately 100 years after the time of Cang Gong, acupuncture had supplanted herbs and moxibustion as the treatment of choice. Only thirteen herbal prescriptions are discussed in the entire *Neijing*. Chapter 55 of the *Suwen* section of the *Neijing* discusses the use of acupuncture for a condition that Cang Gong had treated with moxibustion[15]:

Figure 1.2   Early historical references to acupuncture and related aspects of Chinese culture.

1. One of the earliest known human ancestors, *Homo Erectus*. Fire used for heating, cooking, light, *c.* 500 000–300 000 BC
2. Fire used for healing, *c.* 250 000 BC
3. Previously considered precursor of acupuncture, *c.* 8000 BC
4. Legendary Chinese ancestor and founder of acupuncture, *c.* 2650 BC
5. Legendary manager of flood, *c.* 2000 BC
6. Oracular pronouncements and medical divinations, earliest examples of written Chinese characters, *c.* 1500 BC
7. Earliest book of Chinese philosophy, *c.* 1000 BC
8. Earliest recorded Chinese philosopher, *c.* 725–645 BC
9. Originator of Taoism, *c.* sixth century BC
10. Originator of Confucianism, 551–479 BC
11. Fanmous philosopher and military strategist, author of *Sunzi's Art of War*, *c.* 500 BC
12. Legendary founder of acupuncture, *c.* 407–310 BC
13. Philosopher and follower of Confucius, 385–304 BC
14. Philosopher and follower of Laozi, 369–286 BC
15. Accomplished in 221 BC by Qinshi Huangdi (259–210 BC), the first Qin Emperor
16. One of earliest texts on meridians and moxibustion, *c.* prior to 179 BC
17. Earliest recorded practitioner of acupuncture and moxibustion, *c.* 215–140 BC
18. Includes two earliest known texts on meridians and moxibustion, *c.* prior to 168 BC
19. Oldest existing set of acupuncture needles, *c.* 113 BC; excavated in Hebei Province, 1968
20. Oldest existing model of meridians, *c.* 100 BC; excavated in Sichuan Province, 1993
21. Eminent historian and author of the *Historical Records*, *c.* 135–??? BC
22. Earliest known text on acupuncture and acupoints, *c.* 104–32 BC; includes *Lingshu* and *Suwen*
23. Earliest known text on acupoints, *c.* 32 BC–106 AD
24. Early imperial acupuncturist, *c.* 60–125 AD
25. Practitioner famous for surgery and acupuncture, *c.* 150–208 AD
26. Famous sage of Chinese medicine, *c.* 150–219 AD
27. Acupuncturist and author of *Systematic Classic of Acupuncture and Moxibustion*, *c.* 215–282 AD.

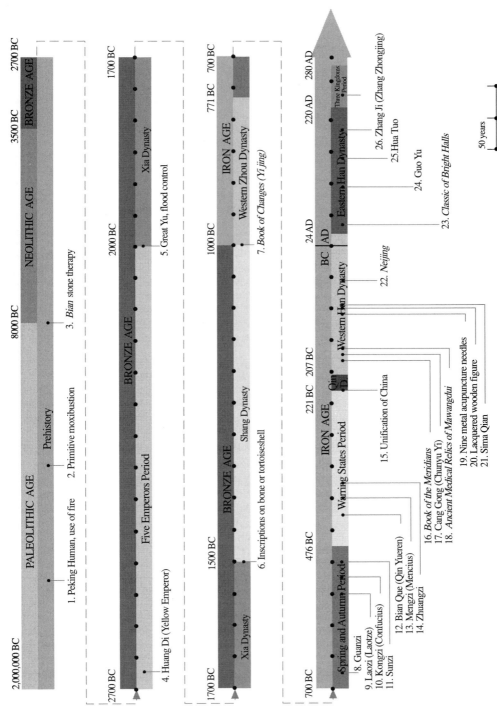

Figure 1.2   Early historical references to acupuncture and related aspects of Chinese culture.

If a patient complains of pain in the lower abdomen accompanied by difficulty in urination and defecation, the condition is called *shan* or abdominal pain, which is due to exposure to cold. One should needle the areas between the lower abdomen and both thighs, as well as the lower back and sacrum. Manipulate the needles until a sensation of heat is induced in the lower abdomen.

The historical evidence discussed above indicates that acupuncture is not as old as has generally been assumed, and that it did not in fact develop gradually since the Neolithic Age (*c.* 8000–3500 BC). Rather, it first appeared late in the Warring States Period (475–221 BC) at the time of Bian Que, developed during the early Western Han Dynasty (206 BC–24 AD) at the time of Cang Gong, and matured during the latter part of the Western Han Dynasty (206 BC–24 AD) at the time of the compilation of the *Neijing* (*c.* 104–32 BC). (See Figure 1.2.)

Was acupuncture invented as the result of repeated empirical experience?

It has been generally believed that acupuncture evolved as a natural outcome of daily life in the Neolithic Age (*c.* 8000–3500 BC), through a process of fortuitous accident and repeated empirical experience. According to this theory, people noticed cases in which physical problems were relieved following an unrelated injury, leading to the discovery of the principle that injury to a certain part of the body can alleviate or even cure a pre-existing disease or disorder in a different part of the body. It is thought that with this discovery, Neolithic Chinese eventually started to use stones, animal bones or pieces of bamboo to induce injury deliberately in order to relieve physical problems. Here is a fictional story describing how this process may have worked[16]:

> Long, long ago a man went to the mountain to cut firewood. Through carelessness his big toe was injured. There was a little bleeding, and his chronic headache by chance disappeared. He paid no attention to this phenomenon at all. His headache recurred later on and was again relieved by accidental injury of his big toe. After the second experience, the man noticed that the relief of his headache might be related to the injury of his toe. Later, whenever his headache recurred, he deliberately injured his big toe and let some blood. Consequently his headache was relieved each time. This is the story of the discovery of the acupoint LR1-Dadun.

If acupuncture did in fact gradually develop through such a process of repeated empirical experience, many similar accounts concerning the discovery of the acupoints and their properties should appear throughout China's 4000 years of recorded history. However, following extensive research I was only able to find one similar example in the immense canon of Chinese medical documents and literature. This case was recorded by Dr Zhang Zihe (*c.* 1156–1228 AD), one of the four eminent physicians of the Jin and Yuan Dynasties (1115–1368 AD), who specialized in bloodletting therapy[17]:

> Bachelor Zhao Zhongwen had an acute eye problem when he went to take part in the imperial examination. His eyes were red and swollen, accompanied by blurred vision and severe pain. He even wanted to die because of the unbearable pain. One day when Zhao was in a teahouse with a friend, a stovepipe suddenly fell and hit him in the forehead, causing a wound about 3–4 *cun* in length and letting copious dark purple blood. The miracle occurred when the bleeding stopped. Zhao's eyes stopped hurting; he could see the road and was able to go home unassisted. The next day he could clearly distinguish the ridge of his roof, and within several days he was completely recovered. This case was cured with no intentional treatment but only accidental trauma.

Actually, the above case at most demonstrates the discovery of bloodletting therapy, which has some essential differences from acupuncture. The point of bloodletting therapy is to take away a certain amount of blood. However, when puncturing the body with solid needles in acupuncture (as differentiated from injecting medicine with a syringe needle), nothing is added to or subtracted from the body.

Bloodletting therapy is universal. Throughout recorded history people around the world have had similar experiences of the beneficial results of accidental injury, and have developed healing methods based on the principle that inducing bleeding in one part of the body can relieve problems in another area. The ancient Greeks and Romans developed venesection and cupping based on the discovery that natural bleeding is beneficial in cases such as fever, headache and disordered menstruation[18]. Europeans during the Middle Ages used bloodletting as a panacea for the prevention and treatment of disease. Detailed directions were given concerning the most favorable days and hours for bloodletting, the correct veins to be tapped, the amount of blood to be taken, and the number of bleedings. Blood was usually taken by opening a vein with a lancet, but sometimes by bloodsucking leeches or with the use of cupping vessels. The procedure was often performed by barbers at public baths[19]. Bloodletting using leeches is still practiced by some doctors in Europe, especially in Germany, as well as by shoemakers in Istanbul. People in Iran habitually let 10–20 drops of blood on the lateral side of the dorsum of the foot (corresponding to the course of the Urinary Bladder Meridian of Foot Taiyang) once a year to prevent the common cold, believing that harmful materials in the blood tend to deposit in the lowest part of the body like deposits in a riverbed, and that bloodletting cleans out this sediment[20].

However, nowhere did these various bloodletting methods develop into a detailed and comprehensive system comparable to that of acupuncture. If acupuncture did indeed arise from repeated empirical experience of accidental injury, it should have developed all over the world rather than just in China. This indicates that repeated experience of accidental injury was not a primary factor in the development of acupuncture.

Did acupuncture using metal needles develop from *bian* stone therapy?

Stone instruments, either natural or worked, were used extensively for hunting and planting in prehistoric times. The use of stone for medical purposes is equally ancient. With the discovery and use of fire during the Paleolithic Age (*c.* 2 000 000–8000 BC), humans discovered that the application of hot stones from their heating and cooking fires could alleviate discomfort. An example of the use of unworked stone to treat disease is recorded in *Therapeutic Methods for 52 Diseases (Wushi' er Bing Fang)*[21]:

> If the hemorrhoid is located on the border of the anus with clinical manifestations of intermittent itching and pain, first excise the hemorrhoid. If the hemorrhoid cannot be excised, mix equal parts of tortoise's brain and [the insect known as] *didan* and apply to the hemorrhoid; then heat a small piece of oval stone, dip it in vinegar, and immediately apply as a compress on the anus. If the condition persists, repeat the treatment several times. This method is efficacious.

With the introduction of stone-working and increasing understanding of disease, Chinese during the Neolithic Age (*c.* 8000–3500 BC) started to chip stones called *bian shi* for medical use. *Bian* stone therapy survived at least until the latter part of the Eastern Han Dynasty (25–220 AD). It is generally assumed that *bian* stone therapy was the precursor of acupuncture using metal needles. This theory holds that Neolithic Chinese had to use stone needles for acupuncture because iron-smelting technology had not yet been developed. Quan Yuanqi, who lived during the Liang Dynasty (502–557 AD), offers the first such interpretation in his annotation of the *Suwen*[22,23]:

> *Bian* stone therapy was an external healing method used in ancient times. Since there was no iron-smelting in antiquity, stone was used to make needles.

This statement indicates that *bian* stone therapy was no longer in use during Quan's time. It also implies that Quan considers the only difference between *bian* stone therapy and acupuncture to lie in the materials used to make the instruments. I believe, however, that there are intrinsic difference between the two therapies.

The ancient definition of the Chinese character *bian* is often used to support the theory that *bian* stone therapy was the direct precursor of acupuncture. The definition given for the character *bian* (砭) in the oldest dictionary of Chinese characters is 'to *ci* (刺) disease with stone'[24]. In contemporary usage, the character *ci* means thorn, or to stab with a thorn-like object. The definition of *bian* is therefore usually given as 'to *needle* or *stab* disease with stone'. This interpretation naturally leads to the association of *bian* stone therapy with acupuncture.

However, I believe that this phrase should be interpreted as 'to *incise* disease with stone', for the following reason. The same dictionary defines *ci* as 'the act of the monarch killing his senior officials'[25]. It is a knife rather than a needle that is used to kill, and 'to kill with a knife' was the primary meaning of *ci* in ancient times. Even today, the term *cike* means a knife-wielding assassin. This indicates that *bian* stones were knife-like rather than needle-like.

Now the question arises as to what kinds of 'diseases' *bian* stones were used to incise. Were they used to treat all diseases, or only certain conditions? References in the ancient documents show that *bian* stone therapy was used specifically to treat *yong* and *ju* conditions (suppurative skin problems such as boils, carbuncles, furuncles etc.)[26].

Yong and *ju* syndromes were common in ancient times, with special chapters on them appearing in both the *Ancient Medical Relics of Mawangdui* and the *Lingshu*[27]. The *Rites of the Zhou Dynasty* refers to a specialized type of surgical practitioner during the Zhou Dynasty (*c.* 1000–256 BC) called *yangyi*, who treated problems such as swollen abscesses, open sores and wounds using *zhuyou* (incantation), medication and incision[28]. Specific treatments appear in the *Ancient Medical Relics of Mawangdui* in sections on *bian* stone therapy and *yong* and *ju* syndromes. The treatment of *yong* and *ju* conditions is divided into presuppurative and postsuppurative stages. *Zhuyou* (incantation), moxibustion and medication, including oral medicine and hot compresses, are employed during the presuppurative stage; *bian* stone therapy is used to drain pus during the postsuppurative stage[29].

The *Ancient Medical Relics of Mawangdui* states that to prevent unwanted side effects when using *bian* stones to drain pus, the size of the stone should be appropriate to the size of the abscess. Four kinds of improper treatment are listed[30]:

> First, to incise a deep abscess superficially is insufficient; second, to incise a shallow abscess deeply is excessive; third, to incise a large abscess with a small *bian* stone is insufficient; fourth, to incise a small abscess with a large *bian* stone is excessive.

The authors of the *Neijing* were obviously very familiar with the history of *bian* stone therapy. They definitively state that *bian* stone therapy originated in eastern China and was used specifically to treat *yong* and *ju* conditions. Chapter 12 of the *Suwen* states[31]:

> The East is the birthplace of heaven and earth. It is close to the sea and teems with fish and salt, so local people eat a lot of fish and prefer a salty flavor. Fish is a hot food;

eating too much fish produces heat in the interior. Salt enters the blood; overeating of salt consumes blood and leads to its slow flow. The combination of interior heat and stagnant blood results in furuncles and sores. Thus people in the east often have dark skin and commonly suffer from swelling abscesses. Accordingly, *bian* stone, an ideal implement for puncturing abscesses, was developed in this area.

Although metal needles, including *feng* (or sharp-edged) and *pi* (or sword) needles, were used to drain abscesses by the time of the *Neijing*, many practitioners still employed *bian* stones for this purpose[32].

Bian stones were designed to be used as surgical knives to drain pus in *yong* and *ju* syndromes. This type of local surgery has nothing in common with acupuncture. If, as previously assumed, *bian* stones were used for acupuncture by Neolithic Chinese solely because they had no worked metal with which to make needles, then acupuncture using metal needles should have replaced *bian* stone therapy as soon as smelting was invented and metal instruments came into widespread use. However, this is not the case. No documents or archeological finds indicate that bronze needles were used medically during the Bronze Age (*c.* 3500–1000 BC).

Iron smelting was invented in China during the Western Zhou Dynasty (*c.* 1000–771 BC), and iron sewing needles made their first appearance during the early Spring and Autumn Period (*c.* 770–476 BC). By the time of *The Ancient Medical Relics of Mawangdui* (*c.* prior to 168 BC), iron instruments including staffs, surgical knives and cauldrons were widely used, and iron was also administered orally as a medicine[33]. However, as previously discussed, no mention of acupuncture using iron needles (or needles of any material) has been found in any document from this time. The earliest reference to the use of metal needles for acupuncture is not found until the *Neijing* (*c.* 104–32 BC), which contains detailed descriptions of nine types of needles, including their shapes and indications. (See Table 1.1 and Figure 1.3.)

In July of 1968, nine metal needles were excavated at Mancheng, Hebei Province, from the tomb of Prince Liu Sheng (???–113 BC) of Zhongshan, elder brother of Emperor Wudi (156–87 BC) of the Western Han Dynasty (206 BC–24 AD). Four of the excavated needles were gold and quite well preserved, while five were silver and had decayed to the extent that it was not possible to restore them completely. (See Figure 1.4.) The number and shapes of the excavated needles indicate that they may have been an exhibit of the nine types of acupuncture needles described in the *Neijing*. This possibility is supported by the fact that a number of additional medical instruments were excavated from the tomb. These included a bronze *yigong* (practitioner's basin), engraved with the Chinese characters *yigong* (practitioner) and used for decocting medicinal herbs or making pills, a bronze sieve used to filter herbal decoctions, and a silver utensil used to pour medicine[34].

Needles have been in use in China since prehistoric times. However, prior to the time of the *Neijing*, their use was limited exclusively to sewing. The original meaning of the Chinese character *zhen*, needle or acupuncture, is a sewing needle[35]. The earliest needles were made of animal bone or bamboo. Many prehistoric bone needles have been unearthed, with presence of an eye indicating that they were used for sewing. Some scholars have inferred that bone needles found with no eye or with points on both ends may have been used by the prehistoric Chinese for medical purposes[36]. However, I believe that it is rash to draw such a conclusion based solely on relics that have lain buried for thousands of years. Rather, it is likely that the eyes of these needles have simply decayed over the millennia.

The historical documents and archaeological evidence discussed above lead me to conclude that *bian* stone therapy was entirely unrelated to the invention of acupuncture,

Table 1.1

Nine metal needles described in the *Neijing* (based on Chapters 1 and 78 of the *Lingshu*)

Name	Modeled on	Length (*cun*)*	Shape	Method and effect	Indications
Chan or plough-share needle	Hairpin, a type of long needle used in ancient times to pin up the hair or attach a hat to the hair	1.6	Large head with sharp tip	Used to prick superficially to clear heat	Sensation of heat in the head or entire body, moving skin problems
Yuan or round needle	Needle used for stitching cotton cloth	1.6	Bamboo tube-shaped body with oval tip	Used to stimulate muscles and expel muscle pathogens	Muscular diseases
Di or arrow-head needle	Stalk of broomcorn millet	3.5	Broomcorn millet-shaped tip	Used to press meridians to invigorate meridian *qi* and expel pathogens	*Qi* deficiency, febrile diseases
Feng or sharp-edged needle	Needle used for stitching cotton cloth	1.6	Bamboo tube-shaped body with sharp three-edged tip	Used to prick collaterals to let blood and clear heat	Febrile diseases, refractory problems, abscesses
Pi or sword needle	Sword-shaped tip	4.0×0.25	Like a sword	Used to incise abscesses to drain pus	*Yong* conditions or abscesses
Yuan-li or rounded sharp needle	Yak tail	1.6	Like a yak tail; small thin body with rounded sharp tip	Used to prick deeply to drain collaterals	Acute diseases, *bi* syndrome, abscesses
Hao or fine needle	Fine long hair	1.6	Fine long body with tip like the proboscis of a mosquito	Used to quicken flow of *qi* and blood; tonify *qi*	Painful *bi* syndrome, deficient patterns
Chang or long needle	Long needle used for sewing	7.0	Like a long sewing needle	Used to quicken flow of *qi* and blood	Deep pathogens, longstanding *bi* syndrome
Da or large needle	Stalk-shaped	4.0	Stalk-shaped body with slightly rounded tip	Used to reduce fluid	Accumulation of fluid in the joints

cun: measurement of length used during the Han Dynasty (206 BC–220 AD). One *cun* is approximately 2.31 cm.

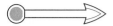

1. *Chan* or plough-share needle

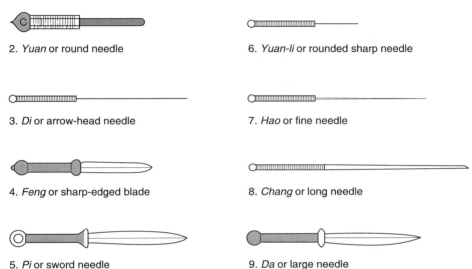

2. *Yuan* or round needle

6. *Yuan-li* or rounded sharp needle

3. *Di* or arrow-head needle

7. *Hao* or fine needle

4. *Feng* or sharp-edged blade

8. *Chang* or long needle

5. *Pi* or sword needle

9. *Da* or large needle

Figure 1.3   Nine metal acupuncture needles, based on Yang Jizhou, *Compendium of Acupuncture and Moxibustion* (1601 AD):

1. *chan* or plough-share needle
2. *yuan* or round needle
3. *di* or arrow-head needle
4. *feng* or sharp-edged needle
5. *pi* or sword needle
6. *yuan-li* or rounded sharp needle
7. *hao* or fine needle
8. *chang* or long needle
9. *da* or large needle.

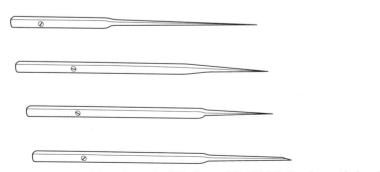

Figure 1.4   Four gold needles excavated from the tomb of Liu Sheng (???–113 BC), based on a black and white photo published in *Archeology* (Wen Wu), 1972, 1: 70–72.

despite the common assumption to the contrary. Incising abscesses to drain pus is not peculiar to ancient Chinese medicine. For instance, Babylonians used bronze knives over 4000 years ago to excise abscesses, yet never developed a system of acupuncture[37]. Furthermore, of the nine acupuncture needles shown in the *Neijing*, three were modeled after sewing needles but none were modeled after *bian* stones. (See Table 1.1.)

In fact, the origin of needles and their applications are two different things entirely. The composition of ancient needles, whether stone, bone, bamboo, bronze or iron, sheds no light on the origins of acupuncture. It is the use rather than the composition of the needle that is important. Needles made of various substances are universal, but only the ancient Chinese were brave enough to needle the body for medical purposes.

Preconditions for the invention of acupuncture

We have demonstrated that the accepted theory that acupuncture originated during China's Late Stone Age (Neolithic Age, *c.* 8000–3500 BC) is incorrect. Let us now attempt to penetrate further the mystery that has veiled this unique healing art since its birth.

Acupuncture appeared quite suddenly on the stage of Chinese history, rather than undergoing a long period of gradual development. Of course, Beijing wasn't built in a day, and the seeds of acupuncture had been bred for centuries before blossoming. Acupuncture arose from a synthesis of ancient knowledge that encompassed flood control, identification of the meridians, knowledge of *qi* and holistic philosophy, all of which were preconditions for its invention.

The first precondition – flood control and understanding of watercourses, the meridians of the Earth

Over 4000 years ago, the Earth started to emerge from the Ice Age. Enormous amounts of ice and snow suddenly melted, and severe flooding was widespread. Such floods occur in the myths and legends of many ancient nations. The story of Noah and the Flood in the Bible is a typical example. The Chinese ancestors living along the Yellow River and the Changjiang (Yangtze) River, the cradle of ancient Chinese civilization, also experienced severe and protracted flooding during this time. Faced with torrential flows, people of almost all other nations considered floods as either punishment from the gods or inescapable and unconquerable calamity[38]. Only the Chinese fought this natural phenomenon.

Among China's numerous legends, the story of how Great Yu controlled the flood is one of the oldest and most popular. It is said that during the Wu Di or Five Emperors Period (*c.* 2700–2000 BC)[39], severe flooding spread over the country and brought great disaster to the people. Gong Gong, the official in charge of water control during the reign of Zhuan Xu (*c.* 2400 BC), was executed because he failed to manage the flood. During the time of the Emperor Yao (*c.* 2200 BC), the flooding continued to wreak great destruction. Emperor Yao appointed his minister Gun to harness the river and control the flood. However, Gun's attempts to obstruct the flood by erecting dikes and dams failed. Gun's son, Yu, was appointed by the next emperor, Shun (*c.* 2100 BC), to continue his father's work. Drawing a lesson from his father's failure, Yu noticed and took advantage of the downward flowing nature of water. He dredged canals according to the physical features of the terrain, to lead the water finally to the sea. After 13 years of hard work, the floods subsided. Because of Yu's great contributions, Emperor Shun abdicated the throne in his favor, and Great Yu established the Xia Dynasty (*c.* 2000–1500 BC).

For thousands of years, Great Yu has been considered not only a hero of flood control but also a model of excellent moral character. It is said that he was so completely dedicated to controlling the waters that for many years he did not visit his wife and children, even when his work took him past the door of his own home. According to the sage Confucius (551–479 BC), Yu passed his house three times without entering it during the course of his labors, and this has led to a popular saying praising those who devote themselves wholeheartedly to their country.

In recognition of Yu's deeds, an essay entitled *Yu's Contribution* was included in China's earliest historical document, the *Shangshu (Classic of History)* (551–479 BC)[40]. The essay records that Yu first divided the country into nine administrative areas according to the mountain chains and watercourses. He then dredged the nine rivers and diked the nine lakes to prevent flooding. This essay is the oldest and most valuable geographical document in China, and is the first exposition of hydrographic networks in the history of Chinese geography.

It may be difficult to separate history from legend in the story of Great Yu controlling the flood, but China's long history of water control is indisputable. The great thinker Guanzi (*c*. 725–645 BC), who lived along the lower reaches of the Yellow and Changjiang (Yangtze) Rivers, said:

Among the five kinds of natural disaster [i.e. flood, drought, wind–fog–hail–frost, pestilence, and plague of insects], flood is the worst.

Guanzi accordingly urged that managing water disasters should take priority, and formulated detailed measures to prevent flood damage[41].

The Chinese ancestors not only recognized the harmful potential of water but also had a deep understanding of its beneficial side. Laozi (*c*. sixth century BC) made the following penetrating observations concerning the character of water:

1. Water is the softest substance on Earth, but it is also the most powerful. It is well known that dripping water can wear through the hardest rock. Needless to say, severe flooding can damage everything in its path.
2. Water is the origin of all living things, including both plants and animals. It gives but never tries to get.
3. Water always flows downward, while people prefer to go upwards.

Laozi concluded that the morality and conduct of the evolved human being should resemble the character of water – that is, one should be steadfast and persevering; bestowing rather than extortive; humble and honest[42].

The ancient Chinese recognized the dual nature of water to both help and harm, and put great effort into turning bane to boon. In their attempts to manage flooding, they paid particular attention to the distribution of watercourses and the valleys in which they were located. *The Classic of Watercourses (Shuijng)*, the world's oldest monograph on watercourses, was compiled by Shang Qin (*c*. first century AD). The book records 137 watercourses, with one chapter devoted to each one. Numerous commentaries have been written on this work. The most famous, *The Annotated Classic of Watercourses (Shuijing Zhu)*, was written by Li Daoyuan (466–527 AD) during the Northern Wei Dynasty (386–534 AD). This book records a total of 1250 watercourses. The British China scholar Dr Joseph Needham noted 'There seems to be no class of geographical literature in Europe quite corresponding to this'[43], indicating that the Chinese ancestors had a special interest in rivers and watercourses.

In addition to the written historical record, the use of advanced water control technology in ancient China can be seen in the Du River Canal (*Dujiang Yan*) in Sichuan

Province, still in use today. Construction of the canal, the most famous water conservancy project of classical China and the entire classical world, commenced during the early Warring States Period (475–221 BC) and was finally completed during the Qin Dynasty (221–207 BC). The canal's uses included water control, irrigation and shipping. This great work of hydraulic engineering continues to play an important role in water control and irrigation to the present day.

The success of the Chinese ancestors in the field of water control heightened their confidence in their dealings with Nature. Most importantly, the principle of dredging rather than diking, first applied to flood control, was extended to social administration and the treatment of human disease. Their understanding of the principle of clearing channels in order to guide a flow, rather than erecting barriers in an attempt to obstruct it, was the first precondition for the birth of acupuncture.

The second precondition – identification of the meridians, from macrocosm to microcosm

Watercourses are the meridians of the Earth in macrocosm. They are the channels that contain the flow of water, the life force of our planet. On the microcosmic scale, the meridians of the human body are the channels that contain the flow of *qi*, the life force of living beings. The identification of the meridians arose directly out of the work of the Chinese ancestors with flood control and watercourses, and was the second precondition for the invention of acupuncture.

Meridian theory provides the theoretical foundation upon which acupuncture is based. However, what is the historical relation of the meridians and acupuncture – which came first? It is generally stated in textbooks of traditional Chinese medicine that the practice of needling preceded the identification of the meridians. It is assumed that the Chinese ancestors first discovered that stimulating their bodies with needles (probably made from *bian* stone in the beginning) could invigorate their energy, or *qi*, and relieve pain and other troubles. Through the ages, they discovered a number of points with specific therapeutic effects. Gradually they linked points with similar effects, 'connecting the dots' as it were, and mapping out the various meridians. According to this scenario, acupuncture was being practiced and the acupoints were being discovered long before the meridians were identified.

However, recent archeological findings challenge this assumption. The excavation in the early 1970s of the *Ancient Medical Relics of Mawangdui* (*c.* prior to 168 BC) opens a window on the status of medicine before the time of the *Neijing* (*c.* 104–32 BC). The most valuable of the *Relics* are two documents concerning meridians, thought to be the oldest extant monographs on meridian theory and moxibustion.

A comparison of the *Ancient Medical Relics of Mawangdui* and the later *Neijing* clearly shows the development of meridian theory from simple to complex and incomplete to complete. (See Table 1.2.) One of the most surprising revelations of the *Ancient Medical Relics of Mawangdui* is that, contrary to general belief, it was moxibustion rather than needling or even *bian* stone therapy that accompanied the early development of meridian theory. Furthermore, moxibustion was applied to the general meridians rather than to discrete points. If, as is generally accepted, needling stimulation did indeed precede and give rise to the identification of the meridians, then references to acupuncture and the acupoints should precede references to the meridians in the ancient documents. However, both the *Ancient Medical Relics of Mawangdui* and additional ancient medical documents excavated at Zhangjiashan in 1983 discuss stimulating the meridians with moxibustion, rather than puncturing discrete points with needles. (See Appendices 2 and 3.)

Table 1.2

Comparison of three classical meridian documents

	Classic of Moxibustion with Eleven Foot-Arm Meridians (c. prior to 168 BC)	*Classic of Moxibustion with Eleven Yin-Yang Meridians* (c. prior to 168 BC)	Chapter 10 of *Lingshu* (c. 104–32 BC)
Title			
Meridians discussed	Eleven of twelve Regular Meridians (Hand Jueyin Meridian not included)	Eleven of twelve Regular Meridians (Hand Jueyin Meridian not included)	Twelve Regular Meridians, fifteen collaterals
Distribution of Meridians	Mainly external; connected organs include heart and liver	Mainly external; connected organs include heart, stomach, and kidney	Twelve Regular Meridians, including both external and internal segments; corresponding twelve *zangfu* organs
Relation among Meridians	Independent	Independent	Interconnected to form a circle
Direction of flow of *qi*	From ends of limbs to trunk and head	Mainly from ends of limbs to trunk and head; Small Intestine and Spleen Meridians from trunk to limbs	Both centripetal and centrifugal
Number of indications	78	147	217
Treatment methods	Moxibustion	No treatment methods mentioned except moxibustion on Foot Shaoyin Meridian	Acupuncture (primary) and moxibustion (secondary)
Remarks	Most basic of the three documents. One group of indications is given for each meridian; use of moxibustion to treat diseases of the general meridian is discussed	Refers to three Hand Yang Meridians, i.e. Large Intestine, San Jiao and Small Intestine, as Tooth Mai, Ear Mai and Shoulder Mai respectively. These names represent the distribution and indications of the meridians. Two groups of indications are given for each meridian	Two groups of indications are given for each meridian. Both style and content are very similar to *Classic of Moxibustion with Eleven Yin-Yang Meridians*

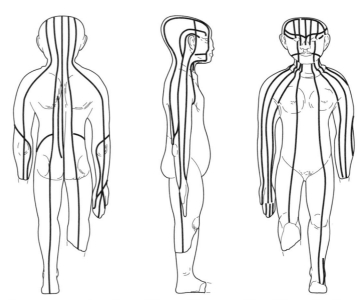

Figure 1.5   Sketch of lacquered wooden meridian model, excavated from Western Han Dynasty tomb (*c*. 100 BC), Mianyang, Sichuan Province in 1993.

A lacquered wooden figure, unearthed in 1993 from a Western Han Dynasty tomb (*c*. 100 BC) located in Mianyang, Sichuan Province, provides further evidence that the identification of the meridians predated the discovery of discrete acupoints. Seventeen red longitudinal lines appear on the figure; two on the front, three on the back, one on each side and five on each arm. (See Figure 1.5.) A comparison of these lines with the meridian pathways described in the *Ancient Relics of Mawangdui* and other early records indicate that the statue is a visual representation of the meridians[44]. The greatest difference between this wooden figure and a much later bronze acupuncture model cast during Northern Song Dynasty (1027 AD) is that the early figure shows only the meridians, while the latter shows both meridians and acupuncture points.

Both ancient documents and archeological findings indicate that identification of the meridians preceded, rather than followed, the invention of acupuncture and discovery of the acupuncture points. (See Chapter 3 for discussion of discovery of the acupoints.) In order to determine how and when the meridians were identified, it is necessary first to consider meridian phenomena.

Meridian phenomena
There are two types of meridian phenomena that occur along the pathways of the meridians; objective meridian manifestations and subjective meridian transmission.

Objective meridian manifestations are visible manifestations along the pathways of the meridians, including pigmentation, pimples, lichenification, bleeding, sweating etc. Some of these manifestations are congenital and normal, and some are acquired and indicate pathological conditions. Acquired manifestations can be either induced or relieved by external stimulation such as needling and moxibustion. Objective meridian manifestations were first recorded in the 1950s by Japanese practitioners[45]. No references to this kind of meridian phenomenon appear in any ancient Chinese medical documents.

Subjective meridian transmission refers to the transmission of sensations along the pathways of the meridians when they are stimulated. The sensations may include soreness, numbness, distension, cold, heat, electric shock or formication. In clinical practice, many people may report localized reactions or various sensations along the meridians. A smaller number experience the transmission of sensations along the entire pathways of the meridians. This kind of meridian phenomenon was first recorded in the *Neijing* (*c.* 104–32 BC). Originally called *qizhi* (arrival of *qi*) or *deqi* (obtaining *qi*), it is now often referred to as *zhengan* (needling sensation).

The phenomenon of arrival of *qi*, or the needling sensation, has received great attention throughout the history of acupuncture. It is the sole criterion for forecasting the effectiveness of acupuncture treatment. There will be good therapeutic results only if needling results in 'arrival of *qi*'. The stronger the needling sensation, the more effective the treatment. The authors of the *Neijing* state[46]:

> The essential point of acupuncture is to induce arrival of *qi*. Treatment will be effective only if there is arrival of *qi*. The effect obtained following arrival of *qi* is visible, just as when a strong wind scatters the last clouds and the overcast sky suddenly becomes fine.

A number of studies on meridian transmission and the phenomenon of arrival of *qi* have been undertaken since the 1950s. In 1950 two Japanese practitioners, Nagahama Yoshio and Maruyama Masao, reported that when they needled a patient with optic atrophy, a strong needling sensation was induced along pathways that were identical to the course of meridians described in the ancient medical literature[47]. Following this report, the number of reports on meridian transmission increased steadily, reaching a peak in the 1970s.

A major study of meridian transmission, involving more than 60 000 subjects, was conducted in China between 1972 and 1978. The *jing* (well) and *yuan* (source) acupoints were stimulated, usually with low frequency pulsating current, to induce transmission. Meridian transmission was considered positive if transmitted sensations were experienced below the wrist or ankle in two meridians, or below the elbow or knee in one meridian. Meridian transmission was considered strongly positive if transmitted sensations were experienced in six or more meridians, or through the entire course of two meridians. Subjects who reported strongly positive meridian transmission were designated meridian-sensitive. The study reported positive meridian transmission in 20.1 per cent of the subjects, and strongly positive meridian transmission in 0.2 per cent of the subjects[48].

The ancient documents indicate an awareness of individual differences in meridian transmission. The *Lingshu* states[49]:

> Because of differences in *qi* and blood, some people experience arrival of *qi* as soon as the needle is inserted, some after manipulation of the needle, some after withdrawal of the needle, and some only after several episodes of needling.

It can be inferred that the Chinese ancestors first became aware of the meridians when they noticed that stimulation could induce transmission of sensation along certain pathways in sensitive people. Recognizing that there was a close relation between transmitted sensations and therapeutic effect, they utilized experimentation and clinical experience to map out these pathways – the meridians – in detail.

What kind of stimulation did the ancient Chinese first apply to induce the phenomenon of meridian transmission? Modern research indicates that moxibustion, acupressure and pulsating current, as well as acupuncture, can all induce meridian transmission[50]. If, as we have demonstrated, the invention of acupuncture and discovery of the acupoints did not occur until well after identification of the meridians, acupuncture can be ruled out as the earliest means of meridian stimulation. Moxibustion is the only type of stimulation discussed in the two oldest texts about the meridians, indicating that moxibustion was the earliest method used to stimulate meridian transmission. This hypothesis is supported by the following points.

Early therapeutic use of moxibustion

The therapeutic use of moxibustion has its roots in the discovery and use of fire by prehistoric humans. Archaeological finds from a number of Early Stone Age (Paleolithic Age, *c.* 2 000 000–8000 BC) sites in China have yielded traces of hearth fires over 500 000 years old. These early Chinese ancestors sat by the fire to roast meat, warm themselves, and hold the night at bay. Gradually they also discovered the therapeutic uses of fire, culminating in the development of moxibustion.

Moxibustion consists of applying a burning substance along the pathways of the meridians in order to stimulate meridian transmission, balance *qi*, and relieve disease and disorder. Actually, 'moxibustion' (burning with moxa) is not an accurate translation of the Chinese medical term for the process *jiu* (to burn). Although the herb moxa (*Artemisiae Argyi Folium*) is the substance most commonly used in moxibustion, numerous other materials were also applied in ancient times. The *Ancient Medical Relics of Mawangdui* mention charcoal, firewood, cattail mat, burlap, rice straw, dry grass, feather and herbs[51].

The earliest use of moxibustion consisted of the application of heat to diseased or general areas, rather than to the meridians or specific acupoints. This primitive and unsystematic therapy can be traced back to remote antiquity. This picturesque description appears in the *Therapeutic Treatments for 52 Diseases*, one of the documents of the *Ancient Medical Relics of Mawangdui*[52]:

> When treating a patient with dysuria, ignite dry grass or firewood. Position the patient's back toward the fire and roast it, while at the same time, two people massage his buttocks. The dysuria can be cured in this way.

A similar treatment for convulsion is recorded in the *Hippocrates*[53]:

> A convulsion must be treated as follows. Keep fires lighted on each side of the bed, and have the patient drink mandrake root to an amount less than would make him delirious; to the posterior tendons apply warm poultices.

Moxibustion is the therapy most frequently mentioned in the *Ancient Medical Relics of Mawangdui* (*c.* prior to 168 BC), and was the primary therapeutic method prior to the popularization of acupuncture around the time of the compilation of the *Neijing* (*c.* 104–32 BC). The *Relics* include two monographs specifically concerned with moxibustion, as well as the *Therapeutic Treatments for 52 Diseases*. Although the *Therapeutic Treatments* is primarily concerned with herbal therapy, moxibustion is also mentioned as a treatment for twenty-three of the fifty-two diseases.

Role of warmth in meridian transmission

Modern research indicates that warming the pathways of the meridians can strengthen meridian transmission. According to one study, meridian transmission is greatly improved if the meridians are warmed for half-an-hour before acupuncture; conversely, meridian transmission is weakened when the pathways are cooled. It is impossible to induce meridian transmission at a room temperature below 15°C, difficult at a room temperature between 15°C and 20°C, and easy at a room temperature above 26°C[54].

The ancient Chinese were aware of this phenomenon, and made full use of it in their practice. Just as cold weather causes water to freeze, so when the body is invaded by external cold or cold is generated in the body due to yang deficiency, the *qi* and blood in the meridians will congeal and the person will suffer from cold limbs. For such a condition, acupuncture alone will be ineffective, no matter how skilled the practitioner is in needling manipulation. Acupuncture cannot soften the congealed meridians, just as a good swimmer cannot swim through ice and a strong digger cannot dig a hole in frozen earth. The correct method in this case is to use heated needles (i.e. heat the tips of the needles until they become red hot prior to needling), or to apply fomentation or hot compresses along the course of the congealed meridians to promote the flow of *qi* and blood, and then needle the meridians for harmonization[55]. The *Neijing* even suggests: 'Do not use acupuncture on cold days, but do not hesitate to puncture if it is warm'[56]. Today, the general principle for treating cold conditions is to apply moxibustion alone or in combination with needling.

The ancient Chinese recognized that puncturing with heated needles can promote the flow of *qi* and blood. They heated needles with fire, or by putting them in the mouth, close to the body or in boiling water[57]. Although warming needles in the mouth might not be acceptable today, heating needles in a more sanitary way is sure to promote the needling sensation and increase effectiveness.

Cooling the head and warming the feet and hands
Cooling the head and warming the feet and hands is an age-old method for preserving good health. People who live in cold climates know that when they go out the first things to get cold are the hands and feet, and when they come in these are the first things they try to warm up. The ancient Chinese offered an excellent explanation for this phenomenon in the *Neijing*[58]:

> Huang Di asked: 'The head is closely connected with the other parts of the body through the bones and tendons. All parts of the body are nourished by the same *qi* and blood. When the weather is cold and the earth is frozen, one's hands and feet become cold, but the face does not feel cold even though it is uncovered. What is the reason?'
>
> Qi Bo answered: 'All the *qi* and blood of the twelve regular meridians and three hundred sixty-five collaterals ascends to the face and orifices. *Qi* vaporizes the body fluid to warm the face, and the face itself has thick skin and is rich in muscles. Therefore, the face is cold-resistant and one does not feel cold on the face even if the weather is very cold.'

The *Nanjing* (*Classic of Difficulties*, *c*. prior to 25 AD), a classic attributed to Bian Que that deals with difficult issues raised in the *Neijing*, gives a further explanation[59]:

> Why is only the face cold-resistant? The reason is that all Yang Meridians converge at the head. All Yin Meridians turn back from the neck and chest, but the Yang Meridians arrive at the head.

According to the principle of Yin and Yang, the upper part of the body (especially the head) is yang and rich in yang *qi*, while the lower part of the body (especially the ends of the extremities) is yin and rich in yin *qi*. In other words, yang *qi* is abundant in the upper portion of the body, but limited in the lower body. This becomes even more apparent when the body's yang *qi* is insufficient. Cold limbs are usually the first signal of yang deficiency.

In accordance with the principle that deficiencies should be supplemented and excesses should be reduced, the ancients believed that adding yang *qi* is beneficial to the lower part of the body (because this supplements a deficiency) but harmful to the upper part of the body (because this would be supplementing an excess). They therefore suggested cooling the head and warming the feet and hands to maintain good health, in this way reducing excess and supplementing deficiency[60].

No specific methods for cooling the head are mentioned in the ancient literature. The reason might be that the head is already in an exposed position, even in the winter and at night. However, many methods for keeping the extremities warm are discussed, including warm clothing, moxibustion, fomentation and massage. Modern studies show that the feet and hands, like the auricle, are miniatures of the body. Warming the feet and hands can therefore promote peripheral blood circulation and influence the functions of the entire body.

Identification of the meridians

We know that moxibustion was practiced long before the identification of meridians, that moxibustion can induce meridian transmission, and that warmth is a major factor in the strength of meridian transmission. It is likely that moxibustion was the earliest method used by the Chinese ancestors to stimulate meridian transmission, harmonization of *qi*, and healing. Based on these points, we may deduce that the therapeutic use of moxibustion led to the identification of the meridians.

The *Ancient Medical Relics of Mawangdui*, as well as other ancient medical documents, discuss the application of moxibustion to the general meridians, mentioning no specific locations. However, this does not mean that moxibustion was applied to the entire meridian. Rather, it is likely that the early use of moxibustion was concentrated on the distal portions of the limbs, according to the principle of cooling the head and warming the feet and hands. This hypothesis is supported by the following points:

- The *Classic of Moxibustion with Eleven Foot-Arm Meridians*, one of the two oldest texts on the meridians from the *Ancient Medical Relics of Mawangdui*, classifies the meridians into Arm and Foot categories. All eleven meridians are described as starting at the distal portion of the limbs and proceeding to the trunk and head[61]. Cang Gong (*c.* 215–140 BC) refers to these originating regions as *maikou*, or mouths of the meridians[62].
- In the first recorded cases of treatment with moxibustion and acupuncture, Cang Gong applied moxibustion to the limbs, rather than the trunk or head, in accordance with the principles of the *Mawangdui* medical documents. He applied moxibustion to left Hand Yangming to treat toothache and to bilateral Foot Jueyin to treat dysuria, and mentions that another practitioner applied moxibustion to the *maikou*, or originating region of Foot Shaoyang in the ankle area, to treat heat in the lungs[63].
- The first acupoints to be discovered were on the limbs. (See Chapter 3 for discussion of discovery of the acupoints.) The earliest mention of acupoints is found in the *Neijing*. Both of its sections, the *Lingshu* and the *Suwen*, contain chapters specifically about the acupoints. The *Lingshu* details acupoints on the limbs, especially specific acupoints below the elbows and knees; while the later *Suwen* concentrates on acupoints on the trunk and head, only mentioning those on the limbs in passing[64]. Since the *Lingshu* is older than the *Suwen*[65], it can be inferred that the ancients first applied stimulation (either moxibustion or needling) to distal portions of the limbs.
- Most acupoints below the elbows and knees, especially the five *shu* (transport) points of each regular meridian, have powerful effects. They are used more frequently for

distal than for local problems. In the two oldest meridians texts from *Mawangdui* (*c.* prior to 168 BC), as well as in Chapter 10 of the *Lingshu* (*c.* 104–32 BC), diseases are attributed to a meridian and its connections. However, by the time of the *Classic of Bright Halls* (*c.* 32 BC–106 AD), the oldest monograph specifically about the acupoints, these problems are attributed to specific acupoints below the elbow and knee. (See Chapter 3 for further discussion of indications of the acupoints.)

☙ Stimulating acupoints on the limbs induces far-reaching meridian transmission. Clinically, every acupuncturist knows that stimulating acupoints on the limbs (especially those below the elbows and knees) generally causes a radiating needling sensation, while acupoints on the trunk and head produce a localized needling sensation. In the study on meridian transmission mentioned above, stimulation was applied to acupoints on the limbs, especially the *yuan* (source) and *jing* (well) acupoints. These are the very points from which the meridians are said to originate in the *Classic of Moxibustion with Eleven Foot-Arm Meridians*. (See Appendices 2 and 3).

These points indicate that the Chinese ancestors first became aware of the existence of the meridians when they applied moxibustion to the extremities, stimulating the phenomenon that came to be called meridian transmission.

Chinese moxibustion vs. Greek cauterization

Why were the meridians identified only in China? The use of heat to treat disease is not peculiar to China, and was used throughout the classical world. The ancient Greeks, for example, made extensive use of fire in their practice. Hippocrates said[66]:

> Those diseases that medicines do not cure are cured by the knife. Those that the knife does not cure are cured by fire. Those that fire does not cure must be considered incurable.

The Greeks considered fire to be the last resort. The following treatment is given for headache[67]:

> If the disease in the head is protracted and intense, and does not go away when the head is cleaned out (by purges), you must either incise the patient's head, or cauterize the vessels all around it. For, of the possible measures that remain, only these offer a hope of recovery.

The Greek application of fire, called cauterization by Hippocrates, is very similar to Chinese moxibustion. The Greeks applied burning raw flax to vessels, diseased areas, and scars, in a process very similar to Chinese suppurative moxibustion[68]. These treatments were quite intense and effective[69]. It is entirely possible that, like their Chinese contemporaries, the Greeks were aware that the application of heat could stimulate meridian transmission. But why did they not mention such a phenomenon? I think the primary reason is that they overlooked the function of *qi* in their practice. The Greeks' understanding of pathology was based on the theory of humors, and the purpose of cauterization was to either block the passage of flux or promote the flow of humors[70]. Humors are visible, so naturally, cauterization was applied to the visible vessels, especially the blood vessels. 'Cauterize the appropriate vessels' is the primary principle in the practice of cauterization[71].

It is true that meridians are often compared to more readily visible structures. Like their Greek contemporaries, the ancient Chinese also initially confused meridians with blood vessels. The *Mawangdui* documents, the oldest monographs on the meridians, refer to the meridians with the term '*mai*', which literally means blood vessels. The *Neijing* classifies the meridians into several types, including *jingmai* or Regular Meridians, *luomai* or collaterals, and *sunmai* or subcollaterals. The ancient Chinese even dissected bodies in an attempt to measure the length and capacity of the Regular Meridians.

Nevertheless, when the ancient Chinese dealt with meridians, they were more interested in what they felt than in what they saw. They focused on the reactions of living bodies rather than anatomical dissections of dead ones. There are two reasons for this. First, *qi* as well as blood flows through the meridians. *Qi* is invisible, and it exists only in the living body. Without the concept of *qi*, the meridians would be identified with the blood vessels, and acupuncture would be synonymous with bleeding therapy. Alternatively, there would be no reason whatsoever to traumatize the body with needles, since acupuncture releases no visible material, such as blood or any other kind of fluid.

The second reason the ancient Chinese focused on invisible *qi* and meridians, rather than visible blood and vessels, might be related to the practice of divination. Early cultures believed the world to be filled with the supernatural, and developed various methods of divination. In ancient China, a special method of divination arose during the Shang Dynasty (*c.* 1500–1000 BC) that had a number of similarities to moxibustion. It consisted of burning animal bones and tortoise shells with moxa or other materials, and predicting the future based on the resulting crackles. Oracular pronouncements were inscribed on the bone or tortoiseshell, and these inscriptions, including divinations concerning disease, have survived as the earliest examples of written Chinese characters.

Although Chinese medicine shook off the bonds of magic long ago, the perspective resulting from the longstanding practice of this type of divination may have contributed to the discovery of the meridians. The shamans who practiced tortoiseshell divination were interested in the distribution of the crackles, rather than the local burned areas. In the same way, early practitioners, also shamans of a sort, were interested in meridian transmission, rather than localized effects[73]. However, they applied fire, in the form of moxibustion, to living bodies in order to stimulate meridian transmission and cure disease, rather than to tortoiseshells in order to stimulate their oracular powers.

To sum up, the meridians are by no means a hypothetical construct developed to link together previously discovered single acupuncture points. Rather, they are special pathways that were identified through the practice of moxibustion and resulting awareness of meridian transmission, combined with the concept of *qi*, and influenced by the practice of divination. Identification of the meridians preceded rather than followed the invention of acupuncture, and provided the second precondition for its development.

The third precondition – recognition and application of *qi*, the fundamental life force

Qi, or life force, is a fundamental term in both traditional Chinese medicine (TCM) and Chinese philosophy. Initially, students of TCM are often confused by this seemingly abstract concept. Actually, the Chinese character for *qi* is quite concrete, originally picturing clouds in the sky. In the early Western Zhou Dynasty (*c.* eleventh century BC– 771 BC) the meaning of the term was extended to include the act of breathing and the substance that is inhaled and exhaled.

Breathing is the most important activity of humans, as well as all other creatures and plants. It is also the most obvious symbol of life. All ancient cultures were aware of this principle, and Hippocrates described it by stating[74]:

> Bodies of men and animals generally are nourished by three kinds of nourishment and
> the names thereof are solid food, drink, and wind. Wind in the body is called breath,

outside it is called air. It is the most powerful of all and it is worthwhile examining its power . . . A man can be deprived of food or drink for two or three days and live, but if the wind passages of the body be cut off, he will die in the brief part of a day, showing that the greatest need of a body is air. Moreover all other activities are intermittent, for life is full of change, but breathing is continuous for all mortal creatures, inspiration and expiration being alternate.

It is recorded in the Hebrew Old Testament that Elijah restored the son of the widow of Zarephath to life by performing artificial respiration[75]. Even animals realize the importance of breath, killing their prey by strangulation or crushing their windpipes.

As breathing is vital to all creatures, it is natural to realize that the substance that we inhale, although invisible, is very important. It is not difficult to understand why the ancestors of many nations considered air to be the origin of all things on earth. The ancient Egyptians held that air was the one constituent of our environment that is of supreme importance – the first power. The air and sun gods were the chief deities of the Greek as well as the Egyptian pantheon – Zeus with his thunderbolts; Apollo, his son, who guided the course of the sun; and Asklepios, the son of Apollo and god of medicine. The Greek philosopher Anaximenes (*c.* 588–524 BC) developed this idea, maintaining[76]: 'Air, taking the form of the soul, imparts life, motion, and thought to animals'.

Integral to the ancient Chinese world view was the recognition of the importance of an invisible material, called *qi*, to life in the universe. The Chinese ancestors believed that the world is made of *qi*, and that the motion of *qi* causes the coming into being, development, and passing away of every thing or phenomenon in the world.

Although the ancient Chinese did not know the composition of what is inhaled and exhaled, they understood that the substance that is inhaled is beneficial to life and the substance that is exhaled is harmful to life. They developed a system of breathing exercises called *tuna* to maintain health and cure disease (*tu* means exhaling and *na* means inhaling). Two main kinds of *tuna* were practiced prior to the Qin Dynasty (221–207 BC). The first was called *shiqi*, or eating *qi*; its purpose was to inhale *qi* of the highest quality[77]. The second was called *zhongxi*, or heel breathing; its purpose was to maximize the inhalation of beneficial (or clear) *qi* and to exhale harmful (or turbid) *qi* as completely as possible[78].

The popular Chinese practice of *qigong* is closely related to *tuna*. *Qigong* is quite recent, gaining widespread popularity only after the liberation of China in 1949. *Gong* means exercise, and *qigong* refers to a series of exercises which utilize *qi* to maintain health and treat disease. Although there are many modern types, *qigong* can best be translated as 'breathing exercises', as this was the earliest type.

It is noteworthy that the first practitioners of breathing exercises were philosophers rather than healers. Laozi, the originator of Taoism, and his follower Zhuangzi (*c.* 369–286) were the first recorded masters of *tuna*[79]. Zhuangzi first defined *tuna* as exhaling the old and inhaling the new, and indicated that deep breathing is beneficial to both health and intelligence[80].

China's ancient healers inherited and developed the idea of *qi* from even earlier philosophers. It is well known that the concept of *qi* is fundamental to traditional Chinese medicine. TCM holds that the combination of earthly and heavenly *qi* gives rise to the birth of the human body, a process of the invisible becoming visible, while dissipation of the combined *qi* leads to death, a process of the visible becoming invisible. Normal life depends upon the unimpeded flow of *qi*; disease and disorder arise from the struggle between *xie qi* (evil *qi*) and *zheng qi* (right *qi*). The purpose of treatment is to strengthen the *zheng qi* and expel the *xie qi*. The concept of *qi* provided the third precondition for the birth of acupuncture.

The fourth precondition – Taoist philosophy and holism

Taoism is China's most ancient school of philosophy and dates back to the time of the legendary Yellow Emperor Huang Di, 2000 years before Christ. Its central concept is the Tao, or Way – the balancing of Yin and Yang (☯), the receptive and active energies of the Universe. Taoism was first expounded as a complete philosophical system in the *Book of Changes*, or *Yijing* (*c.* eleventh century BC). Its precepts were developed by the great philosophers Guanzi (*c.* 725–645 BC) and Laozi (*c.* sixth century BC) during the Spring and Autumn Period (770–476 BC), and matured and flourished during the Warring States Period (475–221 BC), when the free flow of ideas was encouraged by the enlightened State philosophy of 'Let a hundred flowers blossom and a hundred schools of thought contend'.

The success of traditional Chinese medicine owes an immense debt to ancient Chinese philosophy, particularly Taoism with its emphasis on harmonizing the whole. Like their contemporaries the Greeks, the ancient Chinese masters were philosopher-physicians who systematized the knowledge of humanity and Nature handed down across the generations into philosophical doctrines[81]. The encyclopedic *Neijing*, often considered the equivalent of the *Hippocrates*, is the result of this systematization, and lays the foundation for all subsequent Chinese medical literature[82].

Holism, the concept that humanity, society and Nature form an organic unity, and that each part reflects and embodies the whole, is fundamental to Taoism and all other schools of ancient Chinese philosophy[83]. The classical Chinese philosopher-physicians applied and amplified holistic thinking in the field of medicine, where its influence has been comprehensive and profound. It provides not only the framework for traditional Chinese medical theory, but also the working methods for its practice. Humans, the microcosm, are seen as the outgrowth of Nature, the macrocosm. Human and Nature are believed to be similarly constituted and governed by the same laws – 'As above, so below'. Consequently, it is possible to recognize the processes of the human body by observing and analyzing the phenomena of the universe, and the disorders of Human and Nature can be managed using the same principles. This is alluded to in TCM as 'Referring the Human to Heaven and Earth'[84].

Holistic thinking considers that, physiologically, the human body interacts with Nature to form an organic whole and maintain harmony. Pathologically, disorder occurs when either external or internal factors disturb this harmony. Disorder in one organ may affect the others in varying degrees. Diagnostically, the human body is seen as a black box – although it is impossible to observe directly what happens inside, it is possible to deduce the condition inside the body by identifying its outer manifestations. Therapeutically, the purpose of treatment is to cut off the root, or *ben*, (which is inside and invisible) of the problem rather than its manifestation, or *biao*, (which is outside and visible).

Taoist philosophy and the concept of holism provided the fourth and final precondition for the birth of acupuncture.

The invention of acupuncture

The essence of 'Referring the Human to Heaven and Earth' is reasoning by analogy. The invention of acupuncture arose directly from the application of the analogy between the human body and Nature, or microcosm and macrocosm. As has been previously discussed, the ancient Chinese had acquired extensive knowledge about the watercourses of the earth and the meridians of the human body prior to the appearance of acupuncture. Interestingly though, the obvious similarity between these two systems of channels was first recognized by ancient Chinese philosophers rather than by medical practitioners. The great thinker Guanzi (*c.* 725–645 BC) states in the most unequivocal terms: 'Water, the *qi* and blood of the earth, is analogous to [the substance] flowing in the vessels of the human body'[85]. This concept was later adopted by medical practitioners. *Six Pains* (*Liu Tong*) (*c.* prior to 179 BC), one of the ancient medical documents found at Zhangjiashan, states: 'The vessels [meridians] resemble ditches'[86]. The authors of the *Neijing* further developed this analogy. The twelfth chapter of the *Lingshu,* entitled 'Regular Watercourses (*Jingshui*)'[87], deals specifically with the correspondences between the meridians and rivers[88]:

> The twelve Regular Meridians externally correspond to the twelve regular rivers, and internally pertain to and connect with the *zangfu* organs. The rivers carry water and meridians convey blood [and *qi*] . . . [specifically,] Foot Taiyang externally corresponds to the Qing River, and internally pertains to the urinary bladder; Foot Shaoyang externally to the Wei River and internally to the gallbladder; Foot Yangming externally to the Hai River and internally to the stomach; Foot Taiyin externally to the Hu River and internally to the spleen; Foot Shaoyin externally to the Ru River and internally to the kidney; Foot Jueyin externally to the Sheng River and internally to the liver. Hand Taiyang externally corresponds to the Huai River and internally to the small intestine; Hand Shaoyang externally to the Ta River and internally to San Jiao; Hand Yangming externally to the Jiang River [Changjiang or Yangtze] and internally to the large intestine; Hand Taiyin externally to the He River [Yellow River] and internally to the lung; Hand Shaoyin externally to the Ji River and internally to the heart; Hand Jueyin externally to the Zhang River and internally to the pericardium.

The rivers mentioned in the *Lingshu* are located in the basins of the Changjiang (Yangtze) and Yellow Rivers. They can all be found in the early literature on watercourses, and most of them are illustrated on a stone map engraved in 1136 AD. (See Figure 1.1.) It can be seen that the ancient Chinese who compiled this early medical treatise were familiar with the earth's watercourses as well as with the meridians of the human body. They were geographers as well as medical practitioners, and philosophers in their synthesis of Human and Nature – the microcosm and the macrocosm.

Holism considers that since the rivers and meridians are similar in structure, the flow of water in the rivers and the flow of *qi* and blood in the meridians adhere to the same rules. Therefore, their disorders can be similarly managed. If a river course becomes silted up, the water in the river (which by nature flows downward) will overflow. To deal with this condition the river should be dredged rather than diked, in order to guide the water downwards. If a meridian is obstructed, the circulation of *qi* and blood through the meridians will become stagnant and various disorders may occur. To treat this condition, the meridian, like the river, must be dredged. The *Neijing* accordingly states: 'Fine needles should be applied to free the affected meridian and regulate the flow of *qi* and blood'[89].

Conclusions

We may now draw some conclusions about how acupuncture was invented. Upon attaining a thorough understanding of the meridians of human body (the microcosm) and the watercourses of the Earth (the macrocosm), the Chinese ancestors drew an analogy between the two systems of channels. They compared the meridians of the human body to the Earth's rivers, and the *qi* and blood flowing through the meridians to the rivers' waters. Healers of the human body were then able to clear (or dredge) the meridians by puncturing with needles to remove obstructions and promote the flow of *qi* and blood, just as healers of the earth dredged the rivers to remove silt and manage the flood.

Is this deduction correct? Let us now listen to a dialogue between the legendary Chinese Yellow Emperor Huang Di and his Minister, which occurred some time over 2000 years ago[90]:

> Huang Di asked Qi Bo: 'You have told me about the comprehensive nature of *zhendao*, the Tao of Needling. In practice, I adhere to it and believe that it can cure many conditions, even some that had been thought incurable, just as an arrow arrives at its target. Did you obtain your profound knowledge through repeated practice, or by analysis and synthesis of the results of your thorough study of the universe?'
>
> Qi Bo answered: 'When *shengren*, the sages, created the Tao, they had to adhere to certain regulations. Those regulations must conform to the laws of Heaven in their upper aspect, those of Earth in their lower aspect, and those of Humanity in their middle aspect. In this way, they were able to create principles and criteria, which could then be handed down. This is as natural as the fact that a carpenter cannot measure length without a ruler, draw a horizontal line without a straight edge, make a circle without a protractor, or draw a rectangle without a square. The wise follow this principle in their practice. Certainly, this principle is natural, simple, and unchangeable.'
>
> Huang Di asked further: 'I would like to know how the Tao of Needling relates to Nature.'
>
> Qi Bo answered: 'Those versed in the laws of Nature excavate a pond at its lowest point, so that the water within the pond can be drained off and strenuous labor avoided. According to the same logic, they dredge the meridians at the acupoints, the cave-like depressions where *qi* and blood converge. In this way, the meridians can be freed with ease.'

Is this not the answer to the origins of acupuncture, which we have so assiduously sought? The Tao, or Way, is the cardinal concept of Taoism[91]. It primarily refers to the laws of Nature[92]. The 'Unity of Human and Heaven' is one of the primary doctrines of Taoism. Laozi, often considered the founder of Taoism, states: 'Humanity is modeled upon Earth, Earth is modeled upon Heaven, Heaven is modeled upon the Tao, and the Tao is Nature itself'[93]. The ancient Chinese sages, who strove to achieve the synthesis of Taoism, studied the laws of Nature and applied them to both the microcosm and the macrocosm. Healers of the human body were instructed to 'know Heaven above, know Earth below, know Human in the middle'[94]. Believing that humans represent the universe in microcosm, they needled the human body to treat illness in the same way that they dredged the river courses of the Earth to manage the flood. In this way they invented acupuncture, as naturally as water flows downwards.

The invention of acupuncture was based upon natural laws. However, it is by no means natural to treat diseases by needling the body. Frankly speaking, I still sometimes wonder why it was necessary for the ancient Chinese to invent such a traumatic healing way.

Acupuncture and moxibustion both treat disease and disorder by stimulating the flow of *qi* through the meridians, acupuncture with needles and moxibustion with heat. It seems quite reasonable that moxibustion had its first origins in the intuitive application of warmth by prehistoric humans to relieve the pain of injury or disease. Evidence shows that, prior to the invention of acupuncture, therapeutic applications of moxibustion were extensive and successful. Dr Cang Gong's two cases treated with moxibustion effected a cure with just one treatment[95].

The transition from moxibustion to acupuncture was revolutionary. Compared to oxibustion, acupuncture, which uses piercing needles rather than relaxing warmth, is quite traumatic and counterintuitive. Furthermore, the earliest applications of acupuncture were distal rather than local. In other words, the first practitioners of acupuncture created a new healing method that was at the same time traumatic and holistic.

Additional factors

From our modern perspective, it makes no sense to replace a therapeutic method that is safe and comfortable with one that is traumatic and painful. However, this transition did indeed take place, over 2000 years ago! The four preconditions for the invention of acupuncture discussed above were indispensable to the invention of acupuncture, but I believe that further investigation will reveal that the following factors were also instrumental to the process.

Taoism's Law of Paradox, or Contradiction
The Law of Paradox, or Contradiction, is an important doctrine of Taoism. Laozi maintains that every thing or phenomenon has its opposite, and at the point of ultimate development will transform into its reverse. The average person usually recognizes only the superficial or so-called good aspects (e.g. being, happiness, hardness and highness), whereas Laozi emphasizes the deep or so-called bad aspects (e.g. non-being, suffering, softness and lowliness). As non-being gives birth to being, happiness may change into suffering, softness can overcome hardness (as dripping water wears through rock), and lowliness is the basis of highness.

Needling is injurious, but its effect is beneficial. This is a paradox, or contradiction. As Laozi says[96]:

> When one does something harmful, there may be benefit; on the contrary, when one does something beneficial, there may be harm. Other people instruct me, so I will teach others.

With this doctrine in mind, nobody will refuse the minor injury of needling in order to achieve the major benefit of curing disease.

The philosophy of Root and Tip
Root and Tip are translations of the Chinese characters *ben* (本) and *biao* (标); *ben* literally means the root of a tree, and *biao* its tips. As any gardener knows, a tree's branches and leaves will flourish when its roots are well cultivated; conversely, the tips will wither if the root is injured. The ancient Chinese were aware of this natural phenomenon, and developed its essence into the philosophical concept of Root and Tip.

Like Yin and Yang, the concept of Root and Tip is unique to Chinese philosophy and widely applied in traditional Chinese medicine. The principle of Yin and Yang concerns the inter-relatedness of opposites, while the principle of Root and Tip addresses the difference between opposites. When a situation is harmonious, its inherent opposites are in balance and the two aspects of the whole are equal in quantity. Therefore, they can work together with equal effect. However, when a situation is disharmonious, its inherent opposites are out of balance and unequal in quantity, and their effects are unequal. These unequal aspects of the whole can be distinguished into the Root (or principal aspect) and the Tip (or secondary aspect). Just as in the relationship between the root of a tree and its tips, the principal aspect occupies the leading place and determines the onset and development of the secondary aspect.

When addressing a problem, it is necessary to distinguish between the Root and the Tip of the imbalance. Once the Root (or principal aspect) of the problem is solved, the Tip (or secondary aspect) may disappear simultaneously or can be solved with ease. The source of a river is its Root, while its lower reaches are the Tip. Therefore, in the case of flood control it is more important to manage the source of a river than its lower reaches. The meridians, the microcosm of the rivers of the Earth, can also be divided into Root and Tip. Rivers have their source in the mountains, while the meridians have their source at the end of the limbs. According to the *Lingshu*, each Regular Meridian originates at its *jing* (well) acupoint at the end of the limbs, and ends at certain areas of the head, chest or abdomen[97]. Therefore, the section of a meridian located on the limbs is considered to be its Root, while the section on the trunk and head is the Tip. (See Chapter 2 for further discussion of the Root and Tip of the Regular Meridians.) With their deep holistic understanding of flood control and the meridians of the Earth, the ancient Chinese realized that just as managing the source of a river will prevent and control flooding in all its reaches, so stimulating the Root of a meridian on the limb can harmonize disturbances in its corresponding Tip. Following the therapeutic success of applying warmth to general areas of the hands and feet, it was a natural transition to progress to clearing obstructions in the meridians by needling specific acupoints, in the same way that they used tools such as picks and shovels to dredge river courses.

The immediate therapeutic effectiveness of acupuncture

The invention and development of acupuncture was deeply rooted in many aspects of Chinese culture, including technology, geography, philosophy, society and human relations. However, no matter how strong the cultural foundation of acupuncture, it is unimaginable that anyone would continue to experiment with this holistically traumatic and counterintuitive healing method unless it was extremely effective the very first time it was tried. This is indeed the case. The *Historical Records* state that the two cases that Cang Gong treated with acupuncture were cured with just one treatment, and that the treatment was so effective that both patients were reported to be 'fine immediately after needling'. By comparison, although the two cases that Cang Gong treated with moxibustion showed major improvement after one treatment, both cases required further treatment with herbal medicine for 3–6 days. Of the eleven cases he treated solely with herbal medicine, only three were cured with one treatment; the remainder required 2 or more days, with the most intractable cured only after 20 days[98].

The authors of the *Neijing* state that the therapeutic effect of acupuncture is obvious and visible: 'It is just as a strong wind scatters the last clouds and the overcast sky suddenly becomes fine'[99]. Many acupuncture cases discussed in the *Neijing* are said to have achieved a cure immediately upon needling. Almost every practitioner of acupuncture has seen symptoms such as pain and vomiting disappear as soon as the needles are inserted into the body, or within several seconds or minutes. Acupuncture is not only effective but is also simple. Guo Yu (*c.* 60–125 AD), an imperial practitioner of the Eastern Han Dynasty (25–220 AD), is said to have usually achieved a cure by needling just one point[100]. Hua Tuo (*c.* 150–208 AD), another famous surgeon and acupuncturist of the Eastern Han Dynasty, cured many diseases by needling only one or two points[101]. In the clinic, it is common to see cases cured with just one acupoint, one needle and one treatment.

Additional questions concerning the origins of acupuncture

We seem to have lifted the veil covering the origins of acupuncture. However, some points require further clarification.

How did the applications of acupuncture develop?

Clearing the meridians to relieve pain was the first and most obvious use of acupuncture. According to traditional Chinese medicine, the primary pathogenesis of pain is obstruction of the meridians and collaterals[102]. This condition is analogous to overflow of a watercourse. The ancient Chinese deduced that acupuncture can relieve pain by clearing obstructions from the channels of the body, just as the watercourse is cleared by dredging.

The *Neijing* makes reference to the early use of acupuncture to treat *bi* syndrome, one of the most commonly seen pain conditions[103]:

> In the south the weather is hot, the land is low-lying, and fog and mist converge. The local people prefer to eat sour and fermented food and their skin often shows redness. People here usually suffer from spasms and pain in the joints. Thus fine needles, which are suitable for *bi* syndromes, come from the south.

Bi literally means obstruction. According to traditional Chinese medicine, *bi* syndrome, marked by pain in the joints and soreness of the muscles, is caused by external wind, cold, and dampness pathogens, which obstruct the flow of *qi* and blood[104]. Three of the nine types of needles in the *Neijing*, including the filiform needle, which is the main needle used for acupuncture today, were devised to treat *bi* syndrome. (See Table 1.1.)

Not surprisingly, the first use of acupuncture in countries around the world has typically been for pain relief, especially *bi* syndrome.

Although economic and cultural exchange between China and the West via the Silk Road dates back to the invention of acupuncture during the Western Han Dynasty (206 BC–24 AD), acupuncture was not introduced to the West until the seventeenth century. The term acupuncture, or needle puncture, was coined by Willem Ten Rhyne, a Dutch physician who visited Nagasaki, Japan, in the early part of the seventeenth century. In 1683 he published the *Dissertatio de Arthride: mantissa schematica: de Acupunctura* (in Latin), one of the earliest acupuncture documents to appear in the West. In 1810, Dr Berlioz of the Paris Medical School used acupuncture to treat a young woman suffering from abdominal pain. This was the first recorded use of acupuncture in the West. John Churchill, the first known British acupuncturist, published a report in 1821 on the use of acupuncture to treat tympany and rheumatism. John Elliotson, a physician at St Thomas' Hospital in England, published a report in 1827 on forty-two cases of rheumatism treated with acupuncture, and came to the conclusion that this was an acceptable and effective method of treatment for these complaints[105].

Following the initiation of China's reform and opening policy in the 1970s, reports on the use of acupuncture to perform surgery without anesthesia in China started to appear in the Western press. It is not surprising that the first applications of acupuncture in the United States were to induce analgesia or treat pain[106]. Since then, this ancient holistic healing method has received extensive attention from both alternative practitioners and the mainstream medical establishment in the West.

It took approximately 2000 years for acupuncture to spread from the East to the West, and even now in many countries acupuncture is still used solely for pain relief, despite its numerous indications. Acupuncture clinics outside China are often advertised as pain relief clinics, and insurance companies in some countries will only pay for acupuncture when it is used to treat pain. Many people are willing to use acupuncture to relieve pain, even though they may find being punctured with needles extremely traumatic. They can understand the concept of using pain to treat pain, somewhat like being vaccinated with small amounts of toxins to protect against disease. They will tolerate a small pain in order to relieve a greater pain, but wouldn't consider using acupuncture for any of the many other conditions for which it is effective.

How then did acupuncture come to be indicated for disorders other than pain?

> Running water is never stale and a door-hinge never gets worm-eaten. The reason is that they move without cease[107].

This has been a popular Chinese saying concerning maintaining good health since the Qin Dynasty (221–207 BC). According to traditional Chinese medicine, abnormal flow of *qi* and blood is the cause of all ills. *Bi* syndrome (and the pain that accompanies it) is the most typical manifestation of obstructed blood and *qi*, and was the first condition to be treated by acupuncture. However, once the early practitioners realized the effectiveness of acupuncture for pain relief, they speedily applied this new healing method to other conditions.

The number of conditions for which acupuncture was indicated increased rapidly. As mentioned previously, Cang Gong made the first recorded use of acupuncture (*c.* 186–154 BC) during the early part of the Western Han Dynasty (206 BC–24 AD). At this time, herbal treatment was the mainstream of medicine. Only two of Cang Gong's twenty-five recorded cases used acupuncture, but this treatment was so effective that both cases were cured with just one treatment. By the time the *Neijing* (*c.* 104–32 BC) was compiled approximately 100 years later, acupuncture had replaced herbal treatment as the treatment of choice. Both sections of the *Neijing*, the *Suwen* (*Simple Questions*) and the *Lingshu* (*Classic of Acupuncture*), are concerned mainly with the theory and practice of acupuncture; only thirteen herbal prescriptions are mentioned, compared to hundreds of indications for acupuncture. This indicates that the expansion and maturation of acupuncture as a system took only about 100 years[108]. Of course, this expansion continues. Today practitioners and researchers pursue new applications for acupuncture in the treatment of illnesses such as AIDS and addiction syndrome.

The West is currently experiencing an explosive growth in the use of acupuncture, similar to that which occurred in China approximately 2000 years ago. Acupuncture is now being used to treat many other conditions in addition to pain relief, including sequelae of cerebrovascular accident, vomiting, anorexia, irritable colon syndrome, asthma, influenza and other infectious diseases.

Why was the invention of acupuncture unique to China?

The Hippocratic approach of ancient Greece has many similarities to traditional Chinese medicine. Hippocrates, like his Chinese counterparts, was indeed a holist who maintained that Human and Nature combine to form an integrated whole. A Western scholar summarizes[109]:

> Man is related to the environment in which he has evolved and lives, and of an organic balance in the normal body which maintains an equilibrium with all environmental influences of the world and the cosmos; this when disturbed, comes to consciousness as disease and leads to death when reequilibration is no longer possible.

The ancient Greeks, like their Chinese counterparts, also considered pain to be a result of stagnation of blood in the veins, and suggested bleeding to remove the collected blood and relieve pain. Hippocrates points out[110]:

> Bleeding then should be practiced according to these principles. The habit should be ultivated of cutting as far as possible from the places where the pains are wont to occur

and the blood to collect. In this way the change will be least sudden and violent, and you will change the habit so that the blood no longer collects in the same place.

Why did Hippocrates or the ancient Greeks not invent acupuncture or any similar system? I think that there are several answers to this question.

The first reason the ancient Greeks did not invent acupuncture is related to the environment in which they lived. Hippocrates and his predecessors had no knowledge of water control, which as previously discussed is one of the prerequisites for the invention of acupuncture. The ancient Greeks lived on and around islands, and were oriented primarily towards the sea. They were proficient in sailing, and for them (and Mediterranean civilization in general) travel meant travel by sea. It is therefore not surprising that Hippocrates compared physicians to pilots[111]. The Master was fond of analogy, and also compared doctors to various other occupations including iron toolmaker, fuller, cobbler, carpenter, builder, composer, currier, statue-maker, potter, writer and trainer, but nowhere did he mention anything having to do with water control[112]. Certainly the ancient Greeks made no attempt to manage the sea, which remains unconquerable even today.

The second reason that acupuncture did not arise in ancient Greece is that Hippocrates overlooked the practical applications of *qi*. He had an excellent theoretical understanding of *qi* or, in his terms, wind, and maintained that air is the prime necessity for tissue function and that anoxia (or air hunger) is the cause of many diseases[113]. However, this understanding was not carried over into his clinical practice, which was based solely on the theory of humors. According to this theory, the human body is composed of four humors – blood, phlegm, yellow bile and black bile; disturbance of the relative predominance of the humors constitutes disease. Clinically, he classified all diseases into two types: excessive and deficient.

Hippocrates summarized his philosophy as follows: 'Medicine is, in fact, subtraction and addition, subtraction of what is [in] excess and addition of what is wanting'[114]. Various methods of subtraction, usually referred to as 'purges' in the *Hippocrates*, were used in cases of excess[115]. They included bleeding, drugs, exercise and change in the frequency of sexual intercourse. Bloodletting, most frequently used to subtract (or 'purge') the surplus bodily fluid, was accomplished by opening a vein with a lancet, or by cupping[166]. Methods of addition, used in cases of deficiency, included diet, decoctions and exercise.

Blood and other humors, unlike *qi*, are visible, so it was natural for bleeding to become the Hippocratic method of choice for treating disorders of the humors. Although Hippocrates realized the supreme importance of the invisible *qi*, or wind as he called it, he never utilized it in his practice. However, the 'Great Observer' did notice that a great healing force exists in the body, which he called 'Nature'. Hippocrates considered Nature to be inseparable from the constitution (or physical makeup) of the individual. He believed that when the equilibrium of the humors is disturbed, disease results; Nature then makes every effort to restore equilibrium and health[117].

Even the most superficial observer may find an analogy between Hippocrates' 'Nature' and TCM's right *qi*. However, the Chinese and the ancient Greeks approached this natural healing force quite differently. Hippocrates maintains: 'All the physician can do for the patient is to give Nature a chance, to remove by regimen all that may hinder Nature in her beneficent work'[118]. However, his Chinese counterparts exerted their utmost efforts to strengthen this force. Acupuncture is just one of the methods commonly used in TCM[119]. The meridians are needled to invigorate *jing*, or meridian *qi*, and clear obstructions. By activating the flow of *qi* and blood in the meridians, acupuncture can subtract what is excessive and add what is deficient. Were it not for the invisible *qi* that has always been such an integral part of Chinese philosophy, Chinese acupuncture would be synonymous with Greek venesection.

The last reason that the ancient Greeks never invented acupuncture is related to the essentially traumatic nature of acupuncture. As has been previously discussed, needling is traumatic but its effect is beneficial. The ancient Chinese, both practitioners and patients, accepted this paradox willingly because of the Taoist Law of Paradox, or Contradiction. However, Hippocrates, with his holistic thinking, considered that any trauma is injurious, not only to the local area but to the entire body. He states[120]:

> If one injures the smallest part of the body, the whole body actually would experience the disturbance for the very simple reason that the very smallest part actually is composed of the same things as the whole and the single part transmits even the smallest impulse, good or bad, to all other parts that are associated; this because the entire body is integrated with the small parts in pain as well as in pleasure, for the smallest parts (units) transmit to related parts and these again pass on the impulse.

It is apparent from this dogma why Hippocrates invented no therapy as traumatic as acupuncture, with the exception of essential surgical intervention. Although bleeding is also traumatic, Hippocrates considered that cutting the veins to cause bleeding is reasonable because its purpose is to subtract surplus blood or other fluids, which are visible. However, according to Hippocratic holistic thinking, needling the body without letting blood or any other visible fluids is purely traumatic and harmful and is no different from being pricked by a thorn or stung by wasps.

This assumption is also maintained by Douglas Guthrie, a famous medical historian of our era, who suspects that: 'The procedure [acupuncture] probably did more harm than good, though it survives in the treatment of sciatica and fibrositis'[121].

Why was the invention of acupuncture delayed until the Western Han Dynasty (206 BC–24 AD)?

Archeological evidence, including the *Ancient Medical Relics of Mawangdui* (*c.* prior to 168 BC), the documents found at Zhangjiashan (*c.* 187–179 BC), the nine metal acupuncture needles (*c.* 113 BC) discovered in Hebei Province and the lacquered wooden meridian model (*c.* 100 BC) excavated in Sichuan Province, in combination with the contents of the *Neijing* and other early documents, indicates that acupuncture as a fully developed system first emerged during the Western Han Dynasty (206 BC–24 AD), and was marked by compilation of the *Neijing* (*c.* 104–32 BC).

However, we have seen that the conditions necessary for the invention of acupuncture – flood control and understanding of watercourses, identification of the meridians, recognition and application of *qi*, and development of Taoist philosophy and holism – were already in place several hundred years earlier, during or even prior to the Warring States Period (475–221 BC). (See Figure 1.2.) What caused the delay? A historical analysis may provide an answer to this question.

During the Warring States Period (475–221 BC), China consisted of many states, each with its own culture and traditions. For instance, Chinese philosophy developed mainly in the Yellow River basin, especially along the river's lower reaches in the states of Qi and Lu (the present-day Shandong Province). Many eminent philosophers, including Laozi, Confucius, Mencius and Zhuangzi, were from this area. However, many important archeological discoveries concerning the meridians have been found in the Changjiang (Yangtze) River basin, quite a distance from the home of these great philosophers. These include the medical relics found at Mawangdui in Hunan Province and Zhangjiashan in Hubei Province, and the wooden model of the meridians in found in Mianyang, Sichuan Province. These and other finds indicate that recognition of meridians might have been first achieved in the Changjiang (Yangtze) River basin, in the ancient state of Chu (the present-day Hunan Province). (See Figure 1.1.)

Prior to the unification of China in 221 BC by Qinshi Huangdi, the first Qin Emperor, cultural exchange among the states was sluggish or often non-existent due to repeated wars and the barriers of language as well as distance. This lack of communication prevented the synthesis of the various preconditions for the invention of acupuncture that were arising in widely separated areas.

The unification of China by the Qin Dynasty (221–207 BC) laid the foundation for the territorial integration of the diverse states of the Warring States Period. However, culturally speaking this was a period of decadence, stagnation and even decline. The country was dominated by the rigid doctrines of the Legalists[122]. Adherents of all opposing schools of thought were executed or exiled, and almost all non-Legalist books were burned. Although some books survived the burnings, the development of medicine was seriously delayed.

We are fortunate that this dark age in China was much briefer than the Medieval period in Europe. The Great Empire of Qin lasted only 14 years, and was overthrown before all culture was destroyed. The new rulers of the Western Han Dynasty (206 BC–24 AD) learned from the failure of the Qin, and chose the doctrines of Taoism instead of those of the Legalists as their ruling ideology. Politically, Taoism advises rulers to engage in *wuwei*, or non-action. Non-action is not meant literally as 'inactivity', but rather as 'taking no action that is contrary to Nature' – in other words, letting Nature take its own course. This philosophy is completely opposite to that of the Legalists[123].

The adoption of Taoism as the State ideology of the Western Han Dynasty (206 BC–24 AD) not only alleviated class contradictions, but also promoted the development of the natural sciences. The Tao, or Way, the cardinal concept of Taoism, is based on the concept of Yin and Yang (☯), the unity of opposites – the fundamental law of the universe. Also, the Taoist principle of 'Referring the Human to Heaven and Earth' helps people to understand the universe as well as themselves. Ancient China's great achievements in science and technology, especially traditional Chinese medicine, can be attributed to this philosophy.

Taoism lies at the heart of traditional Chinese medicine. Its acceptance during the Western Han Dynasty (206 BC–24 AD) provided the final condition necessary for the birth of acupuncture. During this remote and shadowy era 200 years before the birth of Christ, a group of philosopher-physicians who were dedicated followers of the Tao, as well as industrious practitioners of the healing arts, devoted themselves to the study and systematization of medicine.

The *Neijing* (c. 104–32 BC) was the outcome of this great effort. The close connection between medicine and Taoism is apparent in this book. There are many similarities in both style and spirit between the *Neijing* and other Taoist writings – the *Neijing*, like the *Daodejing*, the essential text of Taoism, has eighty-one chapters[124]; the primary doctrines of Taoism, such as the Tao and Yin and Yang, are found throughout the *Neijing*; the principle of acupuncture is called *zhendao*, or the Tao of Needling; and authorship of the *Neijing*, like many early Taoist books, is attributed to Huang Di, the legendary Yellow Emperor and ancestor of the Chinese people reputed to have lived over 2500 years ago[125]. Just like the medical treatises of the Hippocratic canon, the *Neijing* contains a philosophical element. This medical masterwork is often used as a primary reference for the study of ancient Chinese philosophy, due to its development of the doctrines of Taoism[126].

It may never be known who the authors of the *Neijing* actually were. Despite the loss to history, it was the indifference of these people to fame and fortune, a type of conduct highly appreciated by the Taoists, that made it possible for them to concentrate their minds and create the healing way which has survived until today. These unknown laborers may remain nameless, but their accomplishments will live forever.

The emergence of acupuncture during the Western Han Dynasty (206 BC–24 AD) was not a coincidence. Rather, this miracle was the result of a happy convergence of possibilities and events in China at this precise time in history two millennia ago.

Why has the incorrect theory of the Neolithic origins of acupuncture remained unquestioned?

We are now confronted with a final question. Why has the mistaken theory that acupuncture had its origins in the Late Stone Age (Neolithic Age, *c.* 8000–3500 BC) been accepted so unquestioningly?

A thorough re-evaluation of the evidence confirms that acupuncture is not as old as has generally been assumed, and that it did not in fact develop gradually starting early in the Neolithic Age (*c.* 8000–3500 BC). Rather, this great invention appeared quite suddenly and quickly matured in China approximately two millennia ago, thanks to a particular confluence of many aspects of Chinese culture, including geography, philosophy, society and human relations. However, it seems that scholars of our times have never questioned the general assumptions concerning the origins of acupuncture, despite the contradictions raised by a series of archeological medical finds made since the 1970s. Why have twentieth century scholars been so infatuated with a theory that contains so many errors in logic? Is this only an academic mistake? With further study, it is not surprising to find that there are strong historical reasons.

Political considerations
The renaissance and development of acupuncture in the twentieth century was closely connected with modern China's revolution. During China's War of Resistance against Japan and War of Liberation in the 1930s and 40s, there was a severe lack of doctors practicing Western medicine and dispensing Western medications in the 'liberated areas'. Traditional remedies were widely used because they were cheap, acceptable to the Chinese peasants, and utilized the skills already available in the countryside. In October of 1944, several years before Liberation, Chairman Mao Zedong (1893–1976) summoned practitioners of Western medicine to a meeting on culture and education, to learn from doctors of traditional Chinese medicine in order to serve the broad masses of the people. Subsequently, the government of the Shaanxi–Gansu–Ningxia Border Region convened a forum of Western and traditional Chinese medicine at which the 60-year-old acupuncturist Ren Zuotian described his acupuncture experiences of over 30 years. Many practitioners of Western medicine present at the meeting acknowledged Dr Ren as a master, and indicated a desire to study with him. In April of 1945, the Peace Hospital at Yan'an established clinics for research on acupuncture treatment. In the winter of 1948 the Huabei Medical School was established, with acupuncture as a required course for all students[127]. Following Liberation in 1949, the study and practice of acupuncture gained further momentum. Many hospitals opened acupuncture clinics during the early 1950s, and numerous colleges and institutes were established to teach and investigate acupuncture.

Zhu Lian, the sister of the Chinese People's Liberation Army Commander-in-Chief Zhu De (1886–1976), played a very important role in the spread of acupuncture practice and research during the period prior to and following Liberation. She conducted training courses on acupuncture and moxibustion, and opened acupuncture clinics at a number of hospitals. She published a textbook entitled *New Acupuncture and Moxibustion* in March of 1951, the first of its kind to appear after Liberation. In the book, she reiterated the common belief that acupuncture using metal needles developed from *bian* stone therapy[128]. Even after contradictory archeological evidence was unearthed in the 1970s this idea was never questioned, and articles citing ancient documents and *bian* stone finds continue to be published supporting it[129].

Just as the invention of acupuncture was highly influenced by the State ideology of the Western Han Dynasty (206 BC–24 AD), so the modern interpretation of the origins of acupuncture was deeply influenced by Mao Zedong Thought. As is well known, Mao holds that: 'The masses of the people are the makers of history'. The assumption that acupuncture originated from *bian* stone therapy accords with Mao's concept of history. Whenever stone implements are mentioned, it reminds us of the Stone Age. There were no elite heroes during the Stone Age, only common people, so the association of acupuncture with the Stone Age implies that acupuncture arose from the masses rather than from some elite group or individual. However, a document from the third century AD offers the possibility that acupuncture was invented by an individual. *The Systematic Classic of Acupuncture and Moxibustion*, sometimes translated as *The ABC of Acupuncture and Moxibustion*, states that: 'Huang Di [the Yellow Emperor] created acupuncture using nine needles'[130]. Although Huang Di was a legendary figure, this reference could indicate the existence of an actual individual who at some point was responsible for the creative and intuitive leap that led to the first practice of acupuncture. This archetypal privileged inventor was certainly not a member of the masses, and it is therefore understandable that there has been almost no mention of this possibility in modern China[131].

Philosophical considerations
There is a also a deeper philosophical aspect to the worldwide belief in the prehistoric origins of acupuncture. This is the change in the basic worldview from holism to reductionism.

As has been discussed previously, the idea of the 'Unity of Human and Nature' was the essential philosophical concept of ancient China. This idea permeated almost all aspects of classical Chinese culture, especially traditional Chinese medicine, and the invention of acupuncture arose directly from the application of this holistic thinking. Ancestors of other ancient civilized nations, including India, Greece and Egypt, also held to such holistic thinking in their dealing with the body's health and disease. A contemporary Western scholar comes to the conclusion that[132]:

> Despite their differences in language and metaphors, all of these early cultures approached the body from the same basic worldview. These traditional peoples saw life as an integrated whole, a unity. The body was approached as a unified system in which the physical, mental, and spiritual aspects of life were one. Moreover, each life was united with the life of the universe itself. It is one life, which all things share.

This holistic thinking held sway for very long time. However, the situation has changed since the sixteenth century. Advanced modern science and technology have widened our view of both the microcosm and macrocosm, and have given us a detailed understanding of the human body and Nature at the cellular, molecular, atomic, and even subatomic levels. Unfortunately, we fail to recognize the close relationship among the various parts of the body, and that between the body and Nature, precisely because we have focused too closely on the separate parts. The body is seen as a biochemical machine, consisting of separate components that can be transplanted, replaced or removed if necessary. Moreover, Human and Nature have been separated more completely than ever before. We are surrounded by forests of steel and concrete, and it seems that everything necessary for living is available in supermarkets and malls. The Earth is no longer even considered essential for survival – we think that escape to other heavenly bodies may be feasible by the time the Earth can no longer sustain us.

This basic worldview is known as reductionism. Reductionists attempt to dismantle the world into its component parts and study each part with analytic methods. The theory of the Neolithic origins and empirical development of acupuncture is a typical example of this way of thinking. If modern reductionist scientists were setting out to invent acupuncture today, the process would most likely duplicate the events commonly attributed to the generally accepted theory of its origins. First they would conduct repeated empirical needling experiments (probably starting on animals) to locate acupoints and determine their therapeutic effects. Then they would group together individual points which showed similar effects, and map out connecting lines or meridians. Finally, they would apply this healing way to human beings.

Cultural considerations
Cultural considerations have also contributed to the worldwide acceptance of the incorrect theory of the Neolithic origins of acupuncture. Chinese scholars of acupuncture take great pride in the long history of acupuncture, and think that the older something is, the more authoritative and valuable it is supposed to be. Westerners, by contrast, are infatuated with anything modern – if it is old, it must be outdated and worthless. Consequently a singular phenomenon emerges, where the Chinese make efforts to extend the origins of acupuncture as far back as possible in order to prove its greatness, while Westerners are happy to let this assertion stand unchallenged as a way of denigrating acupuncture. From their perspective, if acupuncture had such vague and primitive origins then it never appeared on the scene as an exciting and innovative new technology, and in fact needn't be considered a technology at all.

Although the ancients, dating back to Quan Yuanqi's annotation of the *Suwen* during the Liang Dynasty (502–557 AD), incorrectly assumed that acupuncture using metal needles developed from *bian* stone therapy, their mistake was superficial. Although they misunderstood the composition of acupuncture needles, they had a strongly holistic outlook, and maintained a holistic perspective in their thinking and practice.

Our mistake, in comparison, is a deep one. In modern society, the Neolithic Age is synonymous with the primitive, the instinctual and the non-technical. We nostalgically attribute the origins of acupuncture to this remote period of prehistory, but we have lost the holistic foundation to which acupuncture owes its existence. Without the foundation of holism, acupuncture becomes no more than a vagrant strand of duckweed, drifting with the current.

Acupuncture as visible holism

A clear picture now emerges of the origins of acupuncture. However, unlike this two-dimensional picture, acupuncture in practice is a holistic sculpture, shaping the flow of *qi* at the interface of the microcosm and macrocosm to heal the human body.

Holism is an abstract concept. It is invisible. Acupuncture, in its integration of Human and Nature, the microcosm and the macrocosm, the physical (the body) and the metaphysical (*qi*), offers a tangible expression of this invisible concept. Acupuncture makes holism visible and concrete. It is nothing less than visible holism.

The central principle of acupuncture calls for needling the lower to cure the upper, and treating the exterior to cure the interior. These treatments are a visible expression of holism. The opposite of this holistic principle would be to treat the head when the head aches and the foot when the foot hurts. A comparison of treatments for toothache and headache by Cang Gong and Hippocrates clearly shows the difference between the two types of therapy. (See Table 1.3.)

Prehistoric trepanning provides another example of non-holistic treatment. This strange surgical operation has engaged the attention of many distinguished archeologists. Evidence of its use has been found in prehistoric skulls from various parts of the world, and the method is still practiced by certain primitive peoples[133]. The practitioners of this operation believed they were casting out a demon that had taken possession of the individual. Such cases of 'devil possession' would today be diagnosed as epilepsy, mental illness, cerebral tumor, migraine etc. As time went on, trepanning came to be employed in cases of fracture of the cranial vault, with this operation employed by Hippocrates.

Table 1.3
Treatment of toothache and headache by Cang Gong and Hippocrates

Ailment	Cang Gong	Hippocrates
Toothache	A senior official of Qi State had tooth decay. Dr Cang applied moxibustion on Hand Yangming of the left side. He also suggested the patient gargle with a decoction of Flavescent Sophora to clean his mouth and kill worms. The cause of the problem was said to be invasion of wind and eating before bed without rinsing the mouth. (From *Historical Records*, 105, 491.)	Pains that arise about the teeth: if the tooth is decayed and loose, remove it; if it is not decayed or loose, but produces pain, dry it out by cautery; medications that are chewed are useful as well. These pains occur when phlegm invades beneath the roots of the teeth; some teeth are decayed by phlegm, others by foods, when they are weak by nature, have caries, and are poorly fixed in the gums. (From *Hippocrates*, Vol. V, *Affections* 4, 13.)
Headache	The Prince of Zichuan had a headache. After examining his pulses, Cang Gong ascertained that the condition was caused by upward movement of yang *qi*, due to the patient lying down with wet hair. In addition to headache, there was also a sensation of heat in the body and restlessness. Dr Cang sprinkled cold water on the patient's head and needled three areas on bilateral Foot Yangming on the lower limbs. The patient was cured immediately. (From *Historical Records*, 105, 491.)	If pains befall the head, it benefits the patient to warm his head by washing it with copious hot water, and to carry off phlegm and mucus by having him sneeze. If, with these measures, he is relieved of his pain, that suffices; but if he is not relieved, clean his head of phlegm, and prescribe a regimen of gruel and drinking water … If, from time to time, pain and dizziness befall the head, the above administrations are also of benefit; it helps, too, if blood is let from the nostrils or from the vessel between the eyes. If the disease in the head is protracted and intense, and does not go away when the head is cleaned out, you must either incise the patient's head, or cauterize the vessels all around it. For, of the possible measures that remain, only these offer a hope of recovery. (From *Hippocrates*, Vol. V, *Affections* 2, 9.)

China, however, is an exception to the worldwide spread of this method of treatment. No archeological relics or documents have been found in China recording the use of such an operation. The reason might be that, thanks to the holistic foundation of traditional Chinese medicine, Chinese healers have always concentrated on the whole rather than the part.

Although acupuncture is just one of many holistic healing systems, it is the only one that offers a visible expression of holism. For instance, Chinese herbal medicine is also holistic; however, what happens inside the body after administration of the herbs is invisible. The actions of the herbs can only be deduced from their curative effects. For instance, flaming upward of the stomach fire may manifest as headache, toothache or even mania. Herbs with cold and purgative properties are therefore administered to cool the stomach fire, in order to relieve headache and toothache and tranquilize mania. This treatment is analogous to taking away firewood from under a cauldron in order to stop it boiling. It is absolutely holistic, but it is not possible to see what is happening inside the body during the course of treatment. By contrast, practitioners of acupuncture will treat the condition by needling ST44-Neiting, a point located on the foot, to cool the stomach fire. The symptoms on the upper part of the body can be relieved effectively through this distal treatment, a visible application of the holistic principle of 'needling the lower to cure the upper'.

Acupuncture is not merely a healing art, but the synthesis and embodiment of thousands of years of Chinese culture. Acupuncturists have the honor of inheriting and practicing not only a system of medicine, but a system of holistic thinking as well.

Notes and References

1. Henry E. Sigerist, *A History of Medicine*, Vol. 1, pp. 115–117. Quoted in Ted J. Kaptchuk, *Chinese Medicine – The Web that has no Weaver*. London: Rider, 1983, p. 109.
2. Wang Benxian, *Foreign Research on the Meridians* (*Guowai Dui Jingluo Wenti De Yanjiu* (国外对经络问题的研究). Beijing: People's Health Press, 1984, p. 260.
3. *Lingshu – The Spiritual Pivot* (*Lingshujing* 灵枢经) (*c.* 104–32 BC). Beijing: People's Health Press, 1963, 9:27. The *Lingshu* states: 'Use the lower to treat the upper; use the upper to treat the lower. Needle the foot to treat the head; needle the popliteal fossa to treat the foot.' The *Lingshu* comprises the first half of the *Neijing – the Yellow Emperor's Inner Classic of Medicine* (*Huang Di Neijing* 黄帝内经) (*c.* 104–32 BC), the seminal work of traditional Chinese medicine.
4. *Encyclopedia Americana*. Danbury: Americana Corporation, 1980, Vol. 1, p. 132.
5. Tom Monte *et al.*, *World Medicine – the East West Guide to Healing Your Body*. New York: G. Putnam & Sons, 1993, p. 38.
6. Cheng Xinnong *et al.*, *Chinese Acupuncture and Moxibustion,* Beijing: Foreign Languages Press, 1987, pp. 1–3.
7. Hebei Medical College, *Collation and Annotation of the Lingshu* (*Lingshujing Jiaozhu* 灵枢经校注) (*c.* 104–32 BC). Beijing: People's Health Press, 1984, Vol. 1, p. 6.
8. Ma Jixing, *Study and Annotation of Ancient Medical Relics of Mawangdui* (*Mawangdui Guyishu Kaoshi* 马王堆古医书考释). Changsha: Human Science and Technology Press, 1992, p. 8.
9. Ma Jixing, *Study and Annotation of Ancient Medical Relics of Mawangdui*, p. 158.
10. *Zhuyou* (祝由), or incantation, was a system of magical or supernatural healing. Ancient beliefs held that disease was caused by invasion of the body by evil spirits or by punishment by the ancestors. A shaman was called upon to pray for pardon, and to cast spells and charms to persuade or force the evil spirit to leave the patient's body. Many ritual *zhuyou* treatments practiced in remote antiquity are preserved in *Therapeutic Methods for 52 Diseases* (one of the

Ancient Medical Relics of Mawangdui). The *Neijing,* written by holists who had shaken off the bonds of magic, includes only a brief introduction to this method (mainly in Chapter 13 of the *Suwen* and Chapter 58 of the *Lingshu*), with no specific techniques given. However, Chapter 13 of the *Suwen* offers the following explanation of the therapeutic mechanism of incantation:

> Huang Di asks: 'I have heard that in the ancient times, when the sages treated, all they had to do was employ methods to guide and change the emotional and spiritual state of a person and redirect the energy flow. The sages utilized a method called *zhuyou*, prayer, ceremony, and shamanism, which healed all conditions . . .'
>
> Qi Bo answers: 'In the ancient times, people lived simply. They hunted, fished, and were with Nature all day. When the weather cooled, they became active to fend off the cold. When the weather heated up in summer, they retreated to cool places. Internally, their emotions were calm and peaceful, and they were without excessive desires. Externally, they did not have the stress of today. They lived without greed and desire, close to Nature. They maintained inner peace and concentration of the mind and spirit. This prevented the pathogens from invading. Even if the pathogens invaded the condition was mild and superficial. Therefore, they did not need herbs to treat their internal state, nor did they need acupuncture [or *bian* stone] to treat the exterior. They simply guided properly the emotions and spirit and redirected the energy flow, using the method of *zhuyou* to heal the condition.'

For details see Maoshing Ni, *The Yellow Emperor's Classic of Medicine*. Boston: Shambhala Publications Inc., 1995, pp. 50–52.
11. It is worth mentioning that many surgical methods preserved in the *Ancient Medical Relics of Mawangdui* and not mentioned in later medical documents may have been in use prior to the Qin Dynasty (221–207 BC). One operation for internal hemorrhoids is very interesting:

> If the venous masses are swollen and obstruct the rectum, kill a dog and cut out its urinary bladder, insert a piece of bamboo tube into the bladder from its lower orifice and tie the bladder to the tube. Put the other end of the bladder into the patient's rectum, blow air into the bladder from the end of the tube with one's mouth to inflate the bladder, then withdraw the expanded bladder slightly to draw the venous masses outside. Cut off the masses slowly and put the powder of scutellaria root (*Scutellariae Radix*) over the diseased area (for antiseptic). Ma Jixing, *Study and Annotation of Ancient Medical Relics of Mawangdui*, p. 524.

12. Sima Qian (*c.* 135 BC–?), *The Historical Records* (*Shi Ji* 史记) (*c.* 100 BC) (eds. Liu Xinglin *et al.*). Beijing: China Friendship Publishing Company, 1994, pp. 486–494. The *Historical Records*, compiled by the great historian Sima Qian (*c.* 135 BC–?), is the first comprehensive Chinese history book. It contains a series of biographies, from the legendary Yellow Emperor Huang Di (*c.* 2650 BC) to the eighth emperor of the Western Han Dynasty, Wu Di (156–87 BC), and is famous for the completeness and accuracy of its contents.
13. Douglas Guthrie, *A History of Medicine*. London and Edinburgh: Thomas Nelson & Sons Ltd, 1946, pp. 56–57. This 40 per cent mortality rate is considerably lower than the 60 per cent mortality rate attributed to Hippocrates in the forty-two cases described in the *Epidemics*.
14. Guo Shiyu, *The History of Chinese Acupuncture and Moxibustion* (*Zhongguo Zhenjiu Shi* 中国针灸史). Tianjin: Tianjin Science and Technology Press, 1989, pp. 68–69.
15. *Suwen (Simple Questions) – the Inner Classic of the Yellow Emperor* (*Huang Di Neijing Suwen* 黄帝内经素问), (*c.* 104–32 BC), annotated by Wang Bing, 762 AD. Beijing: People's Health Press, 1963, 55:286. The *Suwen* comprises the second half of the *Neijing*, the seminal work of traditional Chinese medicine.
16. Sun Yu, *Elementary Knowledge of Formal Logic* (*Xingshi Luoji Jichu Zhishi* 形式逻辑基础知识). Lanzhou: Gansu People's Press, 1980, p. 206.
17. Zhang Zihe (1156–1228 AD), *Confucians' Duties to Their Parents* (*Rumen Shiqin* 儒门事亲). Quoted in *Selection and Annotation of Medical Cases Treated by Past Dynasties' Eminent Acupuncturists* (*Lidai Zhenjiu Mingjia Yian Xuanzhu* 历代针灸名家医案选注) (ed. Li Fufeng). Harbin: Heilongjiang Science and Technology Publishing House, 1985, p. 143.

18. Numerous examples are found in the Hippocratic corpus. 'When in fevers there is deafness, if there be a flow of blood from the nose, or the bowels become disordered, it cures the diseases.' 'When menstruation is suppressed, a flow of blood from the nose is a good sign.' 'When the head aches and the pain is very severe, a flow of pus, water or blood, by the nostrils, ears or mouth, cures the trouble.' *Hippocrates*, eight volumes, English translation by W. H. S. Jones *et al*. Cambridge: Loeb Classical Library, Harvard University Press, 1923, Vol. IV, pp. 151, 167, 183. The quoted version was reprinted in 1995.

19. Roberto Margotta, *The History of Medicine*. New York: Smithmark Publishers, 1996, p. 66.

20. This particular method is not used in traditional Chinese medicine. Although the Iranian treatment calls for puncturing the foot to treat a general condition, the theory is very different from that of Chinese acupuncture.

21. Ma Jixing, *Study and Annotation of Ancient Medical Relics of Mawangdui*, p. 508.

22. Quan's book has been lost since the Southern Song Dynasty (1127–1279 AD). Some excerpts are preserved in the Tang Dynasty (618–907 AD) version of the *Suwen* annotated by Wang Bing in 762 AD. Wang Bing reorganized the entire work and added at least seven chapters of his own. This and the Song Dynasty (960–1279 AD) version, *The Revised and Annotated Inner Classic of the Yellow Emperor: Simple Questions* (*Chongguang Buzhu Huang Di Neijing Suwen* 重广补注黄帝内经素问), annotated by Lin Yi in 1056–1067 AD, are considered the standard versions of the *Suwen*.

23. *Suwen*, 25:161.

24. Xu Shen (*c*. 58–147 AD), *Analytical Dictionary of Characters* (*Shuowen Jiezi* 说文解字) (*c*. 100 AD). Beijing: China Book Company, 1963, p. 195. This is one of the earliest dictionaries of Chinese characters. It was compiled in 100 AD, about 100 years later than the *Neijing*, and discusses the origins of many Chinese characters.

25. *Ibid.*, p. 92.

26. *Yong* (痈) is usually translated as carbuncle and *ju* (疽) as cellulitis. These are two important Chinese medical terms for suppurative skin disorders, equivalent in modern medical terms to suppurative furuncle and acute purulent lymphadenitis.

27. Ma Jixing, *Study and Annotation of Ancient Medical Relics of Mawangdui*, pp. 532–546, 591–600; *Lingshu*, 81:153–155.

28. *Rites of the Zhou Dynasty* (*Zhou Li* 周礼.), written during the Warring States period (475–221 BC), is one of the Confucian classics. It records the official rituals and regulations of the Zhou Dynasty (*c*. 1000–256 BC). Royal doctors at that time were divided into four categories: dieticians, who were responsible for the rulers' food and drink; doctors of internal medicine, who treated diseases and disorders with grains and herbs; surgeons, who treated problems such as swollen abscesses, open sores and wounds using *zhuyou* (incantation), medication and incision; and veterinarians, who treated animals. *The History of Chinese Medicine* (*Zhongguo Yixue Shi* 中国医学史) (ed. Zhen Zhiya *et al*.). Shanghai: Shanghai Science and Technology Press, 1984, 15.

29. Ma Jixing, *Study and Annotation of Ancient Medical Relics of Mawangdui,* pp. 286–291, 591–600.

30. *Ibid.*, pp. 286–290.

31. *Suwen*, 12:80.

32. *Lingshu*, 81:153–155. This chapter is entitled 'Discussion of *Yong* and *Ju*', and is specifically concerned with the treatment of *yong* and *ju* syndromes using *bian* stone.

33. Ma Jixing, *Study and Annotation of Ancient Medical Relics of Mawangdui*, pp. 335, 396, 477, 505, 638.

34. Zhong Yiyan, *Archaeology* (*Kao Gu* 考古), 1972, 3:49–53.

35. Xu Shen, *Analytical Dictionary of Characters*, p. 295.

36. Bai Chun, *Journal of Chinese Medical History* (*Zhonghua Yishi Zazhi* 中华医史杂志), 1993, 23(2): 80.

37. The famous Code of Hammurabi states: 'If the doctor shall treat a gentleman and shall open an abscess with a bronze knife and shall preserve the eye of the patient, he shall receive ten shekels of silver. If the patient is a slave, his master shall pay two shekels of silver'. Douglas Guthrie, *A History of Medicine*, p. 18.

38. Ancient Egypt is an exception. The Nile flooded regularly every year, irrigating and fertilizing the fields on its banks, so the ancient Egyptians benefited from flooding and even prayed for the flood if it did not occur on time.

39. The Wu Di, or Five Emperors Period, refers to the earliest recorded Chinese civilization, around 2700–2000 BC. The five emperors are Huang Di, Zhuan Xu, Di Ku, Yao and Shun.

40. The *Shangshu* (尚书) is the oldest document in Chinese history. It records many important events from the time of Emperor Yao (*c*. 2200 BC) to the Western Zhou Dynasty (*c*. 1000–771 BC). This book is believed to have been compiled by the sage Confucius (551–479 BC).

41. *Guanzi* (*Guanzi* 管子). Beijing: Yanshan Press, 1995, 57:382–389. Guanzi (*c*. 725–645 BC) was one of the great philosophers of the Spring and Autumn Period (770–476 BC). The *Guanzi* is a collection of his ideas and his followers' commentaries, compiled during the Warring States Period (475–221 BC).

42. *Laozi: Annotation and Appreciation of Laozi* (*Laozi Zhushi Ji Pingjie* 老子注释及评介) (ed. Chen Guying). Beijing: China Book Company, 1984, pp. 89, 237, 350. Laozi (Laotze) (*c*. sixth century BC) was one of the great thinkers of the Spring and Autumn Period (770–476 BC), and the originator of Taoism. The *Laozi* (老子), also known as the *Daodejing* (道德经), is a collection of Laozi's ideas and his followers' commentaries, compiled during the early Warring States Period (475–221 BC).

43. Needham Joseph, *Science and Civilization in China*. Cambridge: Cambridge University Press, 1959, Vol. 3, 22:516.

44. He Zhiguo, Study of Western Han Dynasty Lacquered Wooden Figure. *Exploration of Nature* (*Ziran Tansuo* 自然探索), 1995, 14(3):116–121.

45. Wang Benxian, *Foreign Research on the Meridians*. p. 16.

46. *Lingshu*, 1:3.

47. Wang Benxian, *Foreign Research on the Meridians*, p. 1.

48. Li Ding *et al.*, *Meridian Theory* (*Jingluo Xue* 经络学). Shanghai: Shanghai Science and Technology Press, 1984, p. 108.

49. *Lingshu*, 67:123.

50. Li Ding *et al.*, *Meridian Theory*, p. 107; Zhou Meisheng, Research on Meridian Transmission with Moxibustion, *Chinese Acupuncture and Moxibustion* (*Zhongguo Zhenjiu* 中国针灸), 1982, 3:20.

51. Ma Jixing, *Study and Annotation of Ancient Medical Relics of Mawangdui*, pp. 321–653.

52. *Ibid.*, p. 462.

53. *Hippocrates*, Vol. VIII, 79.

54. Li Zhicao *et al.*, *Mystery of Thousands of Years – Research on the Physical Properties of the Meridians* (*Qiangu Zhi Mi – Jingluo Wuli Texing Yanjiu* 千古之迷——经络物理特性研究). Chengdu: Sichuan Educational Press, 1988, pp. 95–97.

55. *Lingshu*, 75:137. The following typical example is recorded in Chapter 6 of the *Lingshu*:

Huang Di asks: 'How should acupuncture be used to treat cold-type *bi* syndrome?'

Bo Gao answers: 'In cases among the common people, apply heated needles. In cases among the royalty, apply herbal fomentation.'

Huang Di asks further: 'How should herbal fomentation be applied?'

Bo Gao answers: 'The herbs used include zanthoxylum (*Zanthoxyli Pericarpium*), dried ginger (*Zingiberis Rhizoma Exsiccatum*), and shaved cinnamon bark (*Cinnamomi Cortex Tubiformis*). The weight of each herb is one *jin* (斤) [unit of weight]. Chew all the herbs into small pieces the size of beans. Put all the herbs into twenty *sheng* (升) [unit of volume] of good wine. Then put one *jin* of cotton and four *zhang* (丈) [unit of length] of fine white cloth into the wine. Seal the container closely with mud. Then put the container into burning horse manure to simmer for five days and nights. Take out the cotton and cloth and dry them in the sun. Then immerse the cotton and cloth in the wine again for twenty hours and then dry them in the sun. Repeat the process until there is no wine in the container. Sew the cloth into six or seven bags six to seven *chi* (尺) [unit of length] long. Put the cotton and dregs into all the bags. Then heat the bags using charcoal made from raw white mulberry. Press the punctured regions with the hot bags to apply heat to the diseased area. Heat the bags again as they cool. Repeat the process thirty times. Apply hot compress whenever needles are used. Cold-type *bi* syndrome can be cured in this way.' *Lingshu*, 6:20.

56. *Suwen*, 26:165.
57. Gao Wu, *Gatherings from Eminent Acupuncturists (Zhenjiu Juying* 针灸聚英) (1529 AD). Shanghai: Shanghai Science and Technology Publishing House, 1961, p. 194.
58. *Lingshu*, 4:11.
59. *Nanjing – the Classic of Difficulties (Nanjing* 难经). Beijing: Scientific and Technological Documents Publishing House, 1996, 47:26. The *Nanjing* (*c.* prior to 25 AD) is an important medical classic compiled after the *Neijing* (*c.* 104–32 BC), sometime during the late Western Han Dynasty (206 BC–24 AD). Its authorship is ascribed to Bian Que, but the real author is unknown. It consists of eighty-one questions and answers dealing with difficult issues raised in the *Neijing*.
60. Ma Jixing, *Study and Annotation of Ancient Medical Relics of Mawangdui*, p. 279.
61. The *Ancient Medical Relics of Mawangdui* include the two earliest extant documents concerning the meridians. They are *The Classic of Moxibustion with Eleven Foot-Arm Meridians* and *The Classic of Moxibustion with Eleven Yin-Yang Meridians*. A comparison of their contents confirms that the first is older than the second. For details see Appendices 2 and 3.
62. *Historical Records*, pp. 486–494.
63. *Ibid.*, pp. 486–494.
64. *Lingshu*, 2:4–8; *Suwen*, 58, 59:291–317.
65. Extensive evidence indicates that the *Lingshu* is older than the *Suwen*. For instance, Chapters 30 and 49 of the *Suwen* are annotations of Chapter 10 of the *Lingshu*; Chapter 54 of the *Suwen* is an annotation of Chapter 1 of the *Lingshu*.
66. *Hippocrates*, Vol. IV, p. 17.
67. *Ibid.*, Vol. V, p. 9.
68. Hippocrates considers suppuration after cauterization to be a good sign. He states:

> When heat causes suppuration, which it does not do in the case of every sore, it is the surest sign of recovery; it softens the skin, makes it thin, removes pain and soothes rigors, convulsions and tetanus. It relieves heaviness of the head. It is particularly useful in fractures of the bones, especially when they are exposed, and most especially in cases of wounds in the head. Also in cases of mortification and sores from cold, of corroding herpes, for the seat, the privy parts, the womb, the bladder – for all these heat is beneficial and conduces to a crisis, while cold is harmful and tends to a fatal tissue. *Hippocrates*, Vol. IV, p. 163.

69. The Greek method of cauterization was terribly traumatic. The *Hippocrates* gives the following treatment for dropsy attributed to a flux in the tissues of the back along the vertebrae:

> Burn three eschars in the tissue of the neck between its vessels, and after you have cauterized, draw the edges of the wound together and make them as flat as possible. *Hippocrates*, Vol. VIII, p. 61.

70. See the Greek treatments for dropsy and sciatica in *Hippocrates*, Vol. VIII, p. 61 and Vol. V, p. 51.
71. *Hippocrates*, Vol. VIII, p. 79.
72. *Lingshu*, 12:41.
73. The history of Chinese medicine can be generally divided into three stages. The first stage, characterized by the use of magic, lasted from before the Shang Dynasty (sixteenth–eleventh centuries BC) until as late as the Western Zhou Dynasty (1000–771 BC). This stage is marked by oracular inscriptions on bones and tortoiseshell, indicating that medical divination was used as the primary form of treatment. The second stage, characterized by the coexistence of magic and medicine, lasted from the Spring and Autumn Period (770–475 BC) until the early part of the Western Han Dynasty (206 BC–24 AD). This stage is marked by the medical documents

from Mawangdui (*c.* prior to 168 BC), which indicate that *zhuyou*, or incantation, was a routine therapy. The third stage, characterized by the separation of magic and medicine, commenced during the middle or latter part of the Western Han Dynasty (206 BC–24 AD). This stage is marked by the compilation of the *Neijing* (*c.* 104–32 BC) and the rapid development of acupuncture.

74. *Hippocrates*, Vol. II, Breaths, p. 3. Quoted in William F. Petersen, *Hippocratic Wisdom*. Springfield: Charles C Thomas, 1946, p. 17.

75. *Bible*, 1 Kings xvii:17–23. Quoted in Douglas Guthrie, *A History of Medicine*, p. 30.

76. H. F. Osborn, *From the Greeks to Darwin*. New York: Macmillan, 1896. Quoted in William F. Petersen, *Hippocratic Wisdom*, p. 227.

77. One of the documents of the *Ancient Medical Relics of Mawangdui* describes this exercise in detail. See Appendix 1.

78. Heel breathing means to inhale deeply and evenly, as if inhaling from the heels instead of the throat. This method is first recorded in Chapter 6 of the *Zhuangzi*, which states: 'The sage breathes deeply. The sage breathes from the heels, while the commoner breathes from the throat'. *Zhuangzi: Brief Annotations of Zhuangzi* (*Zhuangzi Qianzhu* 庄子浅注) (ed. Cao Chuji). Beijing: China Book Company, 1982, 6:88.

79. Wang Buxiong *et al.*, *Developmental History of Chinese Qigong* (*Zhongguo Qigong Xueshu Fazhanshi* 中国气功学术发展史). Changsha: Hunan Science and Technology Publishing House, 1989, p. 27.

80. *Zhuangzi*, 15:227, 6:88.

81. When looking back on the history of philosophy and medicine in China and Greece, corresponding lines of development can be seen in each culture. In Greece, a galaxy of great thinkers preceded Hippocrates, including Thales (624–548 BC), Pythagoras (580–498 BC), Heracleitus (535–475 BC), Empedocles (495–435 BC) and Democritus (*c.* 460–??? BC). Their counterparts in China are Guanzi (*c.* 725–645 BC), Laozi (*c.* sixth century BC), Kongzi (Confucius) (551–479 BC), Sunzi (*c.* contemporary of Confucius) and Mozi (*c.* 475–395 BC). The advanced philosophies that developed on either side of northwestern China's Pamris mountain range, the ancient insurmountable barrier between East and West, led to the almost simultaneous establishment of two great medical systems. Therefore, the following evaluation of the role of Greek philosophy in Greek medicine is also applicable to the role of Chinese philosophy in Chinese medicine:

    It is the work of the early Greek philosophers, however, five hundred years after Homer's day, that Greek medicine is indebted to . . . . . . for that impetus which led men to refuse to be blindly guided by supernatural influences or by rule-of-thumb, and impelled them rather to seek out for themselves the causes and reasons of all the phenomena of Nature. The philosophers, indeed, determined the course which Greek medicine was to take in the hands of Hippocrates and his followers. J. Wright, A medical history on the Timaeus. *Annals of Medical History*, 1925, Vol. viii, p. 116. J. D. Rolleston, The medical aspects of the Greek anthology. *Janus*, 1914, Vol. xix. Quoted in Douglas Guthrie, *A History of Medicine*, pp. 48–49.

82. Despite the many similarities between the *Neijing* and the *Hippocrates*, strictly speaking it is improper to say that they are 'equivalent'. The ancient system of Hippocratic medicine is no longer practiced, and only a few of its fundamental precepts are still considered valid. On the contrary, many of the medical doctrines and healing methods of the *Neijing* are still in use today.

83. Taoism and Confucianism (established by Confucius, 551–479 BC), the two most important Chinese schools of philosophy, both include this doctrine. The difference is that Taoism emphasizes the merging of Human with Nature, while Confucianism strives for the control of Nature by Human.

84. *Lingshu*, 12:41.

85. *Guanzi*, 39:383. The terms vessel (*mai* 脉 in Chinese) and meridian (*jingluo* 经络 in Chinese) were used interchangeably in the *Guanzi* (*c.* 475–221 BC) and other early literature. They were first distinguished from one another in the *Neijing* (*c.* 104–32 BC).

86. Five ancient medical documents (*c.* prior to 179 BC) were unearthed in late 1983 from a Western Han Dynasty (206 BC–24 AD) tomb at Zhangjiashan in Jiangling County, Hubei Province. Three of these documents are identical with *The Classic of Moxibustion with Eleven Yin-Yang Meridians, Methods of Pulse Examination and Bian Stone*, and *Indications of Death on the Yin-Yang Meridians* found at Mawangdui (see Appendix 1). The remaining two documents had never been seen before. *Symptomatology* (*Bingzheng* 病症) is a monograph that discusses a total of sixty-seven symptoms. *Six Pains* (*Liu Tong* 六痛) discusses six types of pain arising from disorders of the bones, tendons, blood, blood vessels, muscles and *qi*. For details, see Gao Dalun, *Collation and Annotation of the Book of Meridians from Zhangjiashan* (*Zhangjiashan Hanjian Maishu Jiaoshi* 张家山汉简脉书校释). Chengdu: Chengdu Press, 1992.

87. The term *jingshui* (经水), or regular watercourses, first appears in the *Guanzi* (*c.* 475–221 BC). Guanzi defines *jingshui* as 'rivers originating in the mountains and finally converging in the sea'. *Guanzi*, 57:383.

88. *Lingshu*, 12:41–42.

89. *Ibid.*, 1:1.

90. *Ibid.*, 38:78.

91. The English term 'Taoism' actually has two different meanings in Chinese. One, *Daojia* (道家) in Chinese, is philosophical. The other, *Daojiao* (道教) in Chinese, is religious. Many Westerners, and even some Chinese, often confuse the two or use them interchangeably. Actually, there are essential differences between the two terms. *Daojia* is China's most ancient school of philosophy, reaching back to the time of the legendary Yellow Emperor, 2000 years before Christ. Its cardinal concept is the Tao – the balancing of Yin and Yang (☯), the receptive and active energies of the Universe. The central writing of Taoist philosophy is the *Laozi*, or *Daodejing*, compiled by the followers of Laozi (*c.* sixth century BC) during the Warring States Period (475–221 BC). *Daojiao* is a native Chinese religion, which appeared hundreds of years later during the late Eastern Han Dynasty (25–220 AD). Taoists (adherents of *Daojiao*) follow the teachings of Laozi, the founder of Taoism (*Daojia*). Here I use the term Taoism to refer to the philosophical *Daojia* rather than the religious *Daojiao*.

92. The Tao (*Dao* 道) encompasses two aspects: the Tao of Substance (*shicunti*), considered to be the origin of all existence and the primordial natural force of the universe, and the Tao of Conduct (*daode*), referring to ethics or morality. A person who achieves Tao embodies the qualities of non-action (*ziran wuwei*), the quietness of the Great Void (*zhixu shoujing*), producing but not having (*sheng er buyou*), gentleness (*rouruo*), modesty (*qianxun*), courtesy (*limao*), diligence (*qinfen*) and thriftiness (*jianpu*). For details on this topic, see *Laozi: Annotation and Appreciation of Laozi*, p. 13.

93. *Laozi: Annotation and Appreciation of Laozi*, 25:163.

94. *Suwen*, 69:402.

95. *Historical Records*, 104:486–494.

96. *Laozi: Annotation and Appreciation of Laozi*, 42:232.

97. *Lingshu*, 5:16.

98. *Historical Records*, 104.

99. *Lingshu*, 1:3.

100. Guo Shiyu, *The History of Chinese Acupuncture and Moxibustion*, p. 78.

101. *Ibid.*, p. 74.

102. *Suwen,* 39:218.

    Huang Di asked, 'I would like to understand pain and its causes'. Qi Bo answered, 'If the *qi* and blood flowing continuously through the body within the channels are attacked by a cold pathogen, they stagnate. If the cold pathogen attacks outside the channels in the periphery, it will simply decrease the blood flow. When it attacks within the channels, it actually blocks the flow of *qi* and blood and causes pain.'

103. *Suwen*, 12:81.

104. *Ibid.*, 43:240.

105. Zhen Zhiya *et al.*, *The History of Chinese Medicine* (*Zhongguo Yixue Shi* 中国医学史). Shanghai: Shanghai Science and Technology Press, 1984, p. 109.

106. Margaret A. Caudill states:

> Early in the 1970s, in the wake of a new politically sanctioned exchange of information between China and the United States, there appeared in the press a number of anecdotal descriptions of surgery without anesthesia being performed in China. A technique called acupuncture was used, whereby slender needles pierced the skin at predetermined foci on the body, the patient being fully awake during the procedure but not feeling the scalpel. Over the next several years this ancient technique of acupuncture enjoyed a brief surge of popularity in the United States, where it was touted by some as a new method to induce analgesia, indeed, as the long-awaited panacea from the Orient ... The evidence now indicates that acupuncture can induce analgesia and that its use is associated with measurable physiological changes. Recent medical reviews show that acupuncture is slowly beginning to be integrated into certain areas of Western Medicine. Quoted in Ted J. Kaptchuk, *Chinese Medicine – The Web that has no Weaver*, p. ix.

107. Ma Jixing, *Study and Annotation of Ancient Medical Relics of Mawangdui*, p. 317.
108. A recent example is the invention and development of auricular therapy. In the 1950s, French doctor Paul Nogier was inspired by the successful treatment of sciatica with cauterization of the auricle to undertake 6 years of further research, culminating in his great discovery of the inverted-fetus shaped distribution pattern of auricular points. He also extended the indications of auricular therapy from pain conditions to many other disorders. Auricular therapy continued to develop for 30 years. See Bai Xinghua *et al.*, *Chinese Auricular Therapy*. Beijing: Scientific and Technical Documents Publishing House, 1994.
109. Hippocrates was holistic in practice as well as theory. He maintains:

> According to my concept of the body there is no beginning, everything is beginning and everything is end, as in a circle. This is true of disease and of the body as a whole ... In order to treat disease we must not only think in terms of the localization which is obvious, but we must treat the organ that is primarily involved. Thereby we can best heal the origin of the disturbance. *De Locis in Homine*, Foes' edition, Ch. 1, Hippocrates. Quoted in William F. Petersen, *Hippocratic Wisdom*, p. 185.

110. *Hippocrates*, Vol. IV, p. 33.
111. Hippocrates states:

> For most physicians seem to me to be the same as bad pilots; the mistakes of the latter are unnoticed so long as they are steering in a calm, but, when a great storm overtakes them with a violent gale, all men realize clearly then that it is their ignorance and blundering which have lost the ship. So also when bad physicians, who comprise the great majority, treat men who are suffering from no serious complaint, so that the greatest blunders would not affect them seriously – such illnesses occur very often, being far more common than serious disease – they are not shown up in their true colors to laymen if their errors are confined to such cases; but when they meet with a severe, violent and dangerous illness, then it is their errors and want of skill are manifest to all. The punishment of the impostor, whether sailor or doctor, is not postponed, but follows speedily. *Hippocrates*, Vol. I, pp. 27–29.

112. *Hippocrates*, Vol. IV, pp. 253–261.
113. Because of the important role of air in normal life, Hippocrates deduces:

> Now I have said that all animals participate largely in the air. So after this I must say that it is likely that maladies occur from this source and from no other. *Hippocrates*, Vol. II, Breaths, 5. Quoted in William F. Petersen, *Hippocratic Wisdom*, p. 17.

114. Hippocrates continues:

> He who performs these acts best is the best physician; he who is farthest removed there from is also farthest removed from the art. *Hippocrates*, Vol. II, Breaths, 1. Quoted in William F. Petersen, *Hippocratic Wisdom*, p. 16.

115. W. H. S. Jones annotates: 'In the *Corpus* "drugs" are purges.' *Hippocrates*, Vol. IV, p. 393: It is interesting to compare the Greek method of 'purging' with the Chinese method of 'dredging'. They reach the same goal by different routes.

116. Hippocrates considered cupping as another important method for drawing excess humors. See *Hippocrates*, Vol. VIII, p. 307. The ancient Greeks and Romans used two kinds of cupping. In wet cupping, superficial incisions were made on the skin, a small piece of burning lint placed in a metal or glass cup, and the cup applied to the skin over the incision. The burning created a vacuum and drew blood from the incision. This process was also known as the artificial leech. In dry cupping, the skin was not cut, but the suction was regarded as sufficient to extract the vicious humor. See Roberto Margotta, *The History of Medicine*. New York: Smithmark Publishers, 1996, p. 71.

117. Tom Monte *et al.*, *World Medicine – the East–West Guide to Healing your Body*, pp. 38–41.

118. *Hippocrates*, Vol. I, p. xvi.

119. Other methods include moxibustion, herbs, diet and *qigong*. One early type of *qigong* was called *shiqi* 食气, or eating *qi*. It consists of breathing exercises to maximize the inhalation of clear, or beneficial, *qi*. This might be an ideal method to treat Hippocrates' air hunger.

120. *De Locis in Homine*. Foes' edition, Ch. 1, Hippocrates. Quoted in William F. Petersen, *Hippocratic Wisdom*, p. 185.

121. Douglas Guthrie, *A History of Medicine*, p. 36.

122. Legalism was an important school of Chinese philosophy that originated during the Spring and Autumn Period (770–476 BC) and was perfected by Han Fei (*c.* 280–233 BC) during the late of Warring States Period (475–221 BC). Han Fei wrote 55 works, which were highly appreciated by Qinshi Huangdi, the First Qin Emperor. Qinshi Huangdi adopted many of Han Fei's ideas as State policy. Politically, the Legalists advocated a system of absolute monarchy. Han Fei advocated the use of violence and wars to seize and consolidate political power, and believed that the Emperor himself should determine all government decrees, criminal laws, and rewards and punishments. Ideologically, the Legalists called for the elimination of those who held different views, in order to establish unity of thinking. Han Fei's ideas played a positive role in the unification of China by Qinshi Huangdi. However, because of its cruel and ferocious persecution of intellectuals as well as the broad masses of the people, the Great Qin Empire lasted only 14 years, and finally was overthrown by a peasant uprising. For details, see the Department of Chinese Philosophical History, Beijing University, *The History of Chinese Philosophy* (*Zhongguo Zhexue Shi* 中国哲学史). Beijing: China Book Company, 1980, Vol. 1, pp. 68–173.

123. Chen Rongjie, *A Source Book of Chinese Philosophy*, p. 136. Quoted in *Laozi: Annotation and Appreciation to Laozi*, p. 67.

124. Nine times nine is eighty-one. Nine is the largest number in Taoist numerology, and eighty-one is the supreme number of the Tao. The *Suwen* and *Lingshu* each consists of eighty-one chapters.

125. Many Taoist scholars of the Warring States Period (475–221 BC) and the early Western Han Dynasty (206 BC–24 AD) attributed their works, such as the *Laozi* and the *Daodejing*, to Huang Di, the semi-mythical Yellow Emperor who was considered to be the founder of Taoism. The *Huainanzi*, a collection of Taoist writings from the Western Han Dynasty (206 BC–24 AD), states: 'Currently, many people have the common view of stressing the past but not the present. So those who develop the doctrines of Tao prefer to attribute authorship of their writings to Shennong [the legendary Chinese emperor and inventor of agriculture] or Huang Di [the Yellow Emperor]'. *Huainanzi* 淮南子. Beijing: Yanshan Press, 1995, 19:512. The authors of the *Neijing* also followed this convention and attributed their own treatises to Huang Di, just as the followers of Hippocrates attributed their writings to Hippocrates.

126. Ren Jiyu, *History of Chinese Philosophy* (*Zhongguo Zhexue Shi* 中国哲学史). Beijing: People's Press, 1966, Vol. 2, pp. 30–36.

127. Zhu Lian, *New Acupuncture and Moxibustion* (*Xin Zhenjiu Xue* 新针灸学). Beijing: People's Press, 1951, 2nd edn, pp. xi–xviii.

128. *Ibid.*, p. 3.

129. Two of the most influential of these articles were written by eminent modern historians Ren Yingqiu and Wang Xuetai, and appeared in the *Fujian Journal of Traditional Chinese Medicine* (*Fujian Zhongyiyao Zazhi* 福建中医药杂志) 1957, 2(6):17–20 and the *Journal of Traditional Chinese Medicine* (*Zhongyi Zazhi* 中医杂志) 1979, 8:59–64 respectively.

130. Huangfu Mi (215–282 AD), *The Systematic Classic of Acupuncture and Moxibustion* (*Zhenjiu Jiayi Jing* 针灸甲乙经) (ed. Huang Longxiang). Beijing: China Medicine and Science Press, 1990, Preface.

131. The influence of Mao's thought on acupuncture was not limited to the interpretation of its origins. Chairman Mao's followers also applied acupuncture as a powerful weapon against Liu Shaoqi's so called revisionist and capitalist line during the Great Cultural Revolution (1966–1976). During this time, a number of acupoints were identified or renamed, including Prevent Revisionism (*Fangxiu* 防修) (1.5 *cun* inferior to SP10-Xuehai), Oppose Revisionism (*Fanxiu* 反修) (4 *cun* above Prevent Revisionism), Criticize Revisionism (*Pixiu* 批修) (1 *cun* inferior to the point midway between the great trochanter and the end of coccyx), and Fight Selfishness (*Dousi* 斗私) (1.5 *cun* posterior and superior to SJ17-Yifeng). *Handbook of New Medical Therapies* (*Xinyi Liaofa Shouce* 新医疗法手册) (ed. Logistics Department of the Kunming Military Area and Revolutionary Committee, Yunnan Province). Kunming: Logistics Department of the Kunming Military Area and Revolutionary Committee, Yunnan Province, 1969.

Also attributed to Chairman Mao is the development of acupuncture anesthesia, considered to be one of the greatest advances in acupuncture in modern times. Acupuncture was first used for anesthesia during the 1950s, and was developed and popularized during the Great Proletarian Cultural Revolution (1966–1976). In 1971, *The People's Daily*, the organ of Chinese Communist Party, reported the discovery of acupuncture anesthesia under a front page banner headline, hailing it as a signal victory of Chairman Mao's proletarian revolutionary line. *People's Daily* (*Renmin Ribao* 人民日报), July 19, 1971:1. Immediately following this report, *Hongqi* (*Red Flag*), the political journal of the party, established a column to discuss the mechanisms of acupuncture anesthesia. See *Red Flag* (*Hongqi Zazhi* 红旗杂志), 1971, 9:58–79; 12:63–70. No other area of the natural sciences received such high-level recognition during this period.

132. Tom Monte *et al.*, *World Medicine – The East–West Guide to Healing Your Body*, p. 7.

133. Douglas Guthrie, *A History of Medicine*, pp. 5–11.

Chapter 2
Meridians – the network of the body

'Meridian theory is the basis of all principles of acupuncture.'
Lingshu

'Meridian' is a translation of the Chinese characters *jingluo*. *Jing* literally means the longitudinal thread in fabric, and refers to the main course of the meridians. *Luo* means to twine or to connect, and refers to the branches of the meridians. The meridians are distributed throughout the body, forming a network that links the upper and lower, and the internal and external, into an organic whole. *Qi* and blood flow through the meridians to nourish the entire body. Meridian theory is fundamental to traditional Chinese medicine, and applications of meridian theory are found throughout the practice of acupuncture. According to the *Lingshu*, 'Meridian theory is the basis of all principles of acupuncture'[1]. This chapter will discuss the primary points and clinical applications of meridian theory.

The system of meridians

The two oldest extant documents concerning the meridians, contained in the *Ancient Medical Relics of Mawangdui* (*c.* prior to 168 BC), discuss only eleven meridians (see Appendices 2 and 3). The *Neijing* (*c.* 104–32 BC) expanded this system to include the twelve Regular Meridians, twelve Divergent Meridians, twelve muscle regions, twelve skin areas, eight Extraordinary Meridians, and fifteen collaterals. The twelve Regular Meridians plus the Ren and Du Extraordinary Meridians are referred to as the Fourteen Meridians, and form the essential portion of the system of meridians.

The twelve Regular Meridians

The twelve Regular Meridians connect internally with the *zangfu* organs and externally with the limbs. Each Regular Meridian has an internal and external segment.

The twelve Regular Meridians are subdivided into six Yin (interior) Meridians and six Yang (exterior) Meridians. These are further subdivided into three Hand and three Foot Yin Meridians, and three Hand and three Foot Yang Meridians. Each Yin (interior) Meridian has a corresponding Yang (exterior) Meridian. The names and interior–exterior (Yin-Yang) relationships of the twelve Regular Meridians are listed in Table 2.1.

Table 2.1
The twelve Regular Meridians and their interior–exterior relations

	Yin Meridians (interior)	*Yang Meridians (exterior)*
Hand	Lung Meridian of Hand Taiyin	Large Intestine Meridian of Hand Yangming
	Pericardium Meridian of Hand Jueyin	San Jiao Meridian of Hand Shaoyang
	Heart Meridian of Hand Shaoyin	Small Intestine Meridian of Hand Taiyang
Foot	Spleen Meridian of Foot Taiyin	Stomach Meridian of Foot Yangming
	Liver Meridian of Foot Jueyin	Gallbladder Meridian of Foot Shaoyang
	Kidney Meridian of Foot Shaoyin	Urinary Bladder Meridian of Foot Taiyang

External segments

The external segments of the Regular Meridians are located on the surface of the limbs, the trunk, the neck and the head. Because there are acupoints distributed along the external segments, they are referred to as 'pathways with acupoints'.

The external segments of the Hand and Foot Yin Meridians are distributed on the inner sides of the arms and legs, in the order of Taiyin, Jueyin, and Shaoyin from anterior to posterior respectively. The external segments of the Hand and Foot Yang Meridians are distributed on the outer sides of the arms and legs, in the order of Yangming, Shaoyang, and Taiyang from anterior to posterior respectively.

The external segments of the three Hand Yang Meridians have relatively short courses, running from the hand to the head. The external segments of the three Foot Yang Meridians cover large areas of the body, stretching from the head to the feet as follows: the Stomach Meridian of Foot Yangming passes through the front of the body, the Gallbladder Meridian of Foot Shaoyang passes through the bilateral sides of the body, and the Urinary Bladder Meridian of Foot Taiyang passes through the back of the body. (See Figure 2.1 a–c.)

Internal segments

The internal segments of the Regular Meridians are located deep within the body. The internal segments have no acupoints, so they are referred to as 'pathways without acupoints'. The internal segment of each Regular Meridian connects with at least two of the twelve *zangfu* organs, i.e. the meridian's related interior *zang* organ and exterior *fu* organ. Each of the six Yang Meridians is connected with and governed by its related exterior *fu* organ, and also connects with its related interior *zang* organ. For example, the Stomach Meridian of Foot Yangming is connected with and governed by the stomach (its related exterior *fu* organ) and also connects with the spleen (its related interior *zang* organ). The six Yin Meridians are governed by and connect with the *zangfu* organs in the opposite way. For instance, the Spleen Meridian of Foot Taiyin is connected with and governed by the spleen (its related interior *zang* organ) and also connects with the stomach (its related exterior *fu* organ).

Connections among the Regular Meridians

The eleven Regular Meridians described in the two oldest meridian texts from Mawangdui (*c.* prior to 168 BC) are said to follow independent pathways, and are not connected with each other. According to these texts, the meridians generally start at the end of the limbs and run inward towards the trunk and head. (See Appendices 2 and 3.) The twelve Regular

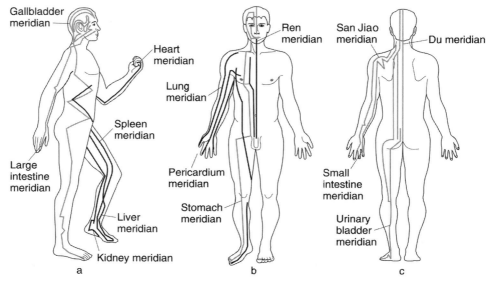

Figure 2.1a–c   General distribution of the Fourteen Meridians:

Lung Meridian of Hand Taiyin
Large Intestine Meridian of Hand Yangming
Stomach Meridian of Foot Yangming
Spleen Meridian of Foot Taiyin
Heart Meridian of Hand Shaoyin
Small Intestine Meridian of Hand Taiyang
Urinary Bladder Meridian of Foot Taiyang
Kidney Meridan of Foot Shaoyin
Pericardium Meridian of Hand Jueyin
San Jiao Meridian of Hand Shaoyang
Gallbladder Meridian of Foot Shaoyang
Liver Meridian of Foot Jueyin
Ren Meridian
Du Meridian.

Meridians described in the *Neijing* (*c.* 104–32 BC), however, are described as connecting with each other at either the head, trunk or limbs to form a circular network. The *Lingshu* describes the layout of this network as follows[2]:

> The three Hand Yin Meridians run from chest to hand, the three Hand Yang Meridians run from hand to head; the three Foot Yang Meridians run from head to foot, and the three Foot Yin Meridians run from foot to abdomen.

According to the *Neijing*, the twelve Regular Meridians connect with each other according to the following principles:

☙ Interior and exterior: Related Yin (interior) and Yang (exterior) Meridians join at the ends of the extremities. For example, the Lung Meridian of Hand Taiyin (Yin, interior) and the Large Intestine Meridian of Hand Yangming (Yang, exterior) join at the tip of the index finger.

☙ Hand and Foot Yang Meridians with the same name join at the head. For example, the Large Intestine Meridian of Hand Yangming (Hand Yangming) and the Stomach Meridian of Foot Yangming (Foot Yangming) join at the nose.

☙ Hand and Foot Yin Meridians join at the trunk, in the thoracic cavity. For example, the Spleen Meridian of Foot Taiyin (a Foot Yin Meridian) and the Heart Meridian of Hand Shaoyin (a Hand Yin Meridian) join at the heart.

The twelve Regular Meridians are thus linked to form a circular system, with *qi* and blood flowing from one meridian to another in succession. This phenomenon is called *liuzhu* – 'flowing and pouring'. *Liu* (flowing) refers to the flow of *qi* and blood within one meridian, and *zhu* (pouring) refers to *qi* and blood pouring from one meridian into the next. Moreover, the flow of *qi* and blood within the meridians is influenced by the sun and the moon, ebbing and flowing in a regular pattern like the tides. This pattern is based on a 24-hour cycle, with each meridian corresponding to one of twelve 2-hour periods. The flow of *qi* and blood in each meridian is greatest each day during the period to which it is related. (See Figure 2.2.) This is the basis for 'Midday–Midnight' acupuncture

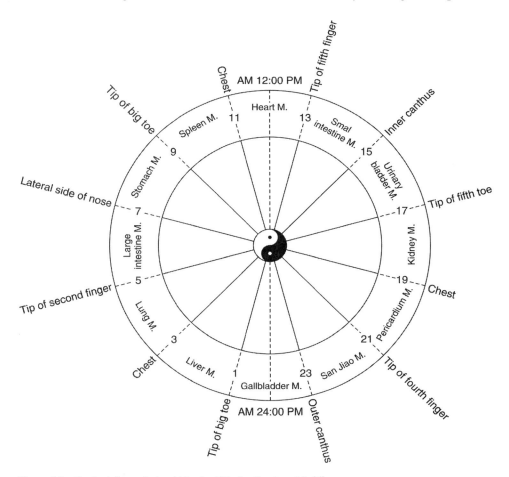

Figure 2.2 Cyclical flow of *qi* and blood within the Fourteen Meridians

treatment, popular during the Jin dynasty (1115–1234 AD). This system called for treating points of a meridian during the period to which it is related. For instance, when treating problems of the Liver Meridian, puncturing should be done between 1 and 3 am, the period at which the flow of *qi* and blood in the Liver meridian is at its peak. (See Chapter 3 for further discussion of Midday–Midnight theory.)

Root and Tip segments of the meridians
The concept of Root and Tip, like that of Yin and Yang, is unique to Chinese philosophy and is widely applied in traditional Chinese medicine. Root and Tip is a crucial principle of meridian theory.

According to both the *Classic of Moxibustion with Eleven Foot-Arm Meridians* from Mawangdui and the *Neijing*, the Regular Meridians originate at the end of the limbs, and end at the head, chest or abdomen. (See Table 2.2.) Each Regular Meridian can therefore be divided into a Root segment, located on the limbs, and a Tip segment, located on the trunk or head. The four limbs are referred to as the four Roots, and the chest, abdomen, and head as the three Tips[3].

Table 2.2
Roots (origins) and Tips (endings) of the six Foot Meridians (based on Chapter 5 of the *Lingshu*)

Meridian	Root (origin)	Tip (ending)
Foot Taiyang	UB67-Zhiyin	Eye
Foot Yangming	ST45-Lidui	Nose and throat
Foot Shaoyang	GB44-Qiaoyin	Ear
Foot Taiyin	SP1-Yinbai	Stomach
Foot Shaoyin	KI1-Yongquan	Root of the tongue
Foot Jueyin	LR1-Dadun	Center of the chest

Although the *Lingshu* gives only the Roots (origins) and Tips (endings) of the six Foot Meridians, the six Hand Meridians follow the same principles of distribution.

Although the flow of *qi* and blood starts at the end of the limbs, these substances are not produced there. In the macrocosm of Nature, water from the sea vaporizes to form rain clouds, which release their waters onto the mountains to form the source of rivers. The rivers carry the water back to the sea, to start the cycle over again. In the microcosm of the human body, the internal *zangfu* organs produce *qi* and blood, which are distributed to the source of the meridians at the end of the limbs. The meridians carry the *qi* and blood to the head and the *zangfu* organs in the chest and abdomen, the sea of the body, to renew the cycle.

Qi and blood circulate ceaselessly through the twelve joined Regular Meridians, nourishing all parts of the body. However, the degree of flow varies in different parts of the meridians, just as the flow of a river varies from its source to the sea. There is relatively little *qi* and blood at the Roots of the meridians at the ends of the limbs, and the amount gradually increases as the meridians approach their Tips at the trunk and head. This increase in flow is reflected in the names of the five types of *shu* (transport) acupoints of the Regular Meridians. Starting at the meridians' points of origin at the ends of the limbs and progressing towards the elbows and knees, these are the *jing* (well), *ying* (spring), *shu* (stream), *jing* (river) and *he* (sea) acupoints respectively. (See Figure 2.3.)

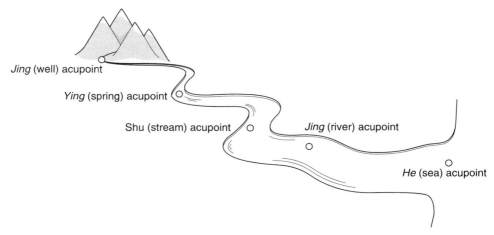

Figure 2.3 Illustration of five types of *shu* (transport) acupoints:

jing (well) acupoint
ying (spring) acupoint
shu (stream) acupoint
jing (river) acupoint
he (sea) acupoint

The distinction between the Root and Tip segments of the twelve Regular Meridians is highly significant. Each Regular Meridian is like a tree. Just as cultivating the roots of a tree will enable its branches and leaves to flourish, stimulating the Root of a meridian can harmonize disturbances in its Tip. This is one of the essential principles of acupuncture. The *Neijing* states[4]:

> The core of nine needle therapy is the theory of Root and Tip, or the origins and endings of the meridians. If this theory is grasped, the essentials of acupuncture may be expressed in one sentence. If not, the Tao of Needling will be lost completely.

The powerful effect of the acupoints on the limbs, especially those below the elbows and knees, provides convincing supporting evidence for this theory. (See Chapter 3 for discussion of the various acupoints.)

The twelve Divergent Meridians

The twelve Divergent Meridians are major branches of the twelve Regular Meridians. Each Regular Meridian has a corresponding Divergent Meridian. They are located deep within the body, and have no acupoints on their pathways.

Principles of distribution

The Divergent Meridians adhere to the following principles of distribution:

- Divergence: most Divergent Meridians split off from their Regular Meridians around the elbows and knees. There are no specific acupoints at the points of divergence.
- Entrance: all of the Divergent Meridians enter either the thoracic or abdominal cavities to connect with their related *zangfu* organs. For example, the Stomach Divergent Meridian enters the abdominal cavity to connect with the stomach (its related exterior

fu organ) and the spleen (its related interior *zang* organ). Additionally, the three Foot Yang Divergent Meridians connect with the heart, as well as with their related *zangfu* organs.

❧ Emergence: all Divergent Meridians emerge from the upper thoracic cavity, and then ascend to the neck or head.

❧ Convergence: after emerging from the thoracic cavity, the six Yang Divergent Meridians converge with their Regular Meridians, while the six Yin Divergent Meridians converge with their Regular Meridians' related Yang Regular Meridians. For example, the Large Intestine Divergent Meridian, a Yang Divergent Meridian, converges with the Large Intestine Meridian. However, the Lung Divergent Meridian, a Yin Divergent Meridian, does not converge with the Lung Meridian, but rather with the Large Intestine Meridian, the Lung Meridian's related Yang Regular Meridian.

Table 2.3 shows the general distribution of the twelve Divergent Meridians.

Functions of the Divergent Meridians

The twelve Regular Meridians resemble primary river courses, while the Divergent Meridians are their major tributaries. Although the Divergent Meridians do not have their own acupoints, they fulfill the following functions:

❧ They strengthen the connection between related Yin (interior) and Yang (exterior) Regular Meridians, through the convergence of the Yin Divergent Meridians with their Regular Meridians' related Yang Meridians.

❧ They strengthen the connection between the Regular Meridians and their related *zangfu* organs, by entering the thoracic or abdominal cavities and connecting with their Regular Meridians' related *zangfu* organs.

❧ They provide an indirect connection between the Yin Meridians and the head. Unlike the Yang Regular Meridians, the Yin Regular Meridians, with the exception of the Liver Meridian, do not end at the head. Rather, they are indirectly linked with the head via the connection between their Divergent Meridians and their related Yang Regular Meridians.

❧ They strengthen the connection between the Foot Yang Meridians and the heart. The three Foot Yang Meridians do not connect with the heart directly, but their Divergent Meridians establish such a connection.

Briefly, the Divergent Meridians extend the scope of distribution and expand the therapeutic indications of their Regular Meridians. For example, the Divergent Meridian of the Urinary Bladder Meridian of Foot Taiyang connects with the anus, so some acupoints of the Urinary Bladder Meridian are effective for diseases of the anus.

The twelve muscle regions

The muscles and tendons of the body are divided into twelve regions according to the distribution of the twelve Regular Meridians. The muscles and tendons along the pathway of each meridian are considered to be that meridian's muscle region. For example, the muscles and tendons along the pathway of the Lung Meridian are called the Lung Meridian muscle region.

Each muscle region originates at the end of the limbs and ascends to the trunk and head, attaching to the joints and bones along the way. Although some muscle regions enter the body cavities, they have no physical connections with the internal *zangfu* organs[5].

Table 2.3

General distribution of the twelve Divergent Meridians (based on Chapter 11 of the *Lingshu*)

Meridian	Divergence	Entrance	Emergence	Convergence
Lung Divergent Meridian	Diverges from Lung Meridian above elbow	Connects with lungs and large intestine	Connects with throat	Converges with Large Intestine Meridian
Large Intestine Divergent Meridian	Diverges above elbow, connects with shoulder and back of neck	Connects with lungs and large intestine	Connects with throat	Converges with Large Intestine Meridian
Stomach Divergent Meridian	Diverges above knee	Connects with stomach, spleen and heart	Follows throat, connects with mouth and eyes	Converges with Stomach Meridian
Spleen Divergent Meridian	Diverges above knee	Connects with stomach, spleen and heart	Connects with throat and root of tongue	Converges with Stomach Meridian
Heart Divergent Meridian	Diverges above elbow	Connects with heart	Runs along throat, disperses through face	Converges with Small Intestine Meridian at inner canthus
Small Intestine Divergent Meridian	Diverges at shoulder joint	Connects with small intestine and heart		
Urinary Bladder Divergent Meridian	Diverges from popliteal fossa, connects with anus	Connects with the urinary bladder, kidney, and heart	Runs along back of the neck	Converges with Urinary Bladder Meridian
Kidney Divergent Meridian	Diverges from popliteal fossa	Connects with kidney	Meets with Dai Meridian and root of tongue	Converges with Urinary Bladder Meridian at back of neck
Pericardium Divergent Meridian	Diverges above elbow	Connects with San Jiao	Runs along throat and posterior portion of ear	Converges with San Jiao Meridian at mastoid region
San Jiao Divergent Meridian	Diverges from main course at head, arrives at vertex (DU20-Baihui)	Connects with San Jiao and pericardium		
Gallbladder Divergent Meridian	Diverges at thigh, distributes around external genital region	Connects with gallbladder, liver and heart	Runs along throat, disperses over face, connects with eyes	Converges with Gallbladder Meridian at outer canthus
Liver Divergent Meridian	Diverges at dorsum of foot, joins Gallbladder Divergent Meridian at external genital region			

The muscle regions are nourished by the *qi* and blood flowing through the meridians. They function to stabilize the joints and maintain normal range of movement.

Disorders of the muscle regions include *bi* (obstruction) syndrome, contracture, stiffness, spasm and muscular atrophy. There is usually tenderness in the affected areas. These tender points determine the location of acupoints that should be stimulated.

The twelve skin regions

The skin, as well as the muscles and tendons, is divided into twelve regions according to the distribution of the twelve Regular Meridians. The skin over the pathway of a meridian is considered to be that meridian's skin region. For example, the skin along the pathway of the Lung Meridian is called the Lung Meridian skin region.

The meridians connect internally with the *zangfu* organs and diffuse externally to the skin, providing lines of communication between the interior and exterior of the body. When the interior of the body is out of order, positive signs will usually manifest on the skin region of the affected meridian. These manifestations may include pimples, eminences or changes in skin color, and can help identify the internal situation. Therapeutically, stimulating the skin regions can harmonize the interior disturbance. Methods may include acupoint compresses, sand scraping and cupping.

Extraordinary Meridians

In addition to the twelve Regular Meridians, there are eight Extraordinary Meridians. They are the Du, Ren, Chong, Dai, Yangqiao, Yinqiao, Yangwei, and Yinwei Meridians. The Ren and Du Meridians are generally classified with the twelve Regular Meridians, with these Fourteen Meridians constituting the principal part of the meridian system. The eight Extraordinary Meridians are as follows.

- The Du Meridian: *du* means to supervise and urge. The Du Meridian, also translated as the Governing Vessel, runs vertically along the midline of the back, a yang area of the body. It connects with all of the Yang Regular Meridians at DU14-Dazhui. The Du Meridian is therefore referred to as the 'Sea of all Yang Meridians', and functions to govern the flow of *qi* and blood in the Yang Meridians.
- The Ren Meridian: *ren* means to control or nourish. The Ren Meridian, also translated as the Conception Vessel, runs vertically along the midline of the front of the body, which has yin properties. It connects either directly or indirectly with all of the Yin Meridians, and is therefore referred to as the 'Sea of all Yin Meridians'. It functions to control the flow of *qi* and blood in the Yin Meridians. The Ren Meridian originates inside the lower abdomen, the location of the uterus in the female and the *jinggong*, or Palace of Essence, in the male. The *qi* and blood of this meridian nourish the fetus.
- The Chong Meridian: *chong* means communications hub. The Chong Meridian, also translated as the Penetrating Vessel, is related to the Stomach Meridian of Foot Yangming and the Kidney Meridian of Foot Shaoyin, the acquired and congenital foundations of the body respectively. The Chong Meridian therefore connects acquired and congenital *qi* and blood. It is referred to as the 'Sea of the Twelve Regular Meridians', and serves as their communications hub.
- The Dai Meridian: *dai* means belt. The Dai Meridian originates in the hypochondriac region and encircles the waist like a girdle. It functions to hold in place all the meridians that pass through the trunk.

☯ The Yangqiao and Yinqiao Meridians: *qiao* means to walk on tiptoe. The Yangqiao and Yinqiao Meridians originate from the depressions below the outer and inner sides of the ankle joint respectively. They function to regulate motion of the lower limbs. Their points of origin, UB60-Kunlun and KI6-Zhaohai, are applied for treatment of strephenopodia, strephexopodia and foot drop. Additionally, the two meridians meet at the inner canthus and then enter the skull to connect with the brain. They therefore function to regulate the closing and opening of the eyes – in other words, dominate awakening and falling asleep. When *qi* in the Yangqiao Meridian is excessive, it will be difficult to close the eyes at night, resulting in insomnia. Conversely, when *qi* in the Yinqiao Meridian is excessive, it will be difficult to keep the eyes open during the day, resulting in drowsiness.

☯ The Yangwei and Yinwei Meridians: *wei* means to maintain. The Yangwei Meridian originates at UB63-Jinmen, and ascends to intersect with the Small Intestine Meridian of Hand Taiyang, the San Jiao Meridian of Hand Shaoyang, and the Du Meridian (which connects with all the Yang Regular Meridians). The Yangwei Meridian therefore functions to maintain all the Yang Regular Meridians. The Yinwei Meridian starts from KI9-Zhubin, and ascends to intersect the Spleen Meridian of Foot Taiyin, the Liver Meridian of Foot Jueyin, and the Ren Meridian (which connects with all the Yin Regular Meridians). The Yinwei Meridian therefore functions to maintain all the Yin Regular Meridians.

The eight Extraordinary Meridians differ from the twelve Regular Meridians in the following respects.

Time of identification
The Extraordinary Meridians were identified later than the Regular Meridians. The Regular Meridians (with the exception of the Pericardium Meridian) were first mentioned in the medical documents from Mawangdui (*c.* prior to 168 BC), and further systematized in the *Neijing* (*c.* 104–32 BC). A limited discussion of the Ren, Du and Chong Meridians appears in the *Neijing*, and a description of the distribution of all eight Extraordinary Meridians appears in the *Nanjing* (*c.* 32 BC–220 AD). However, a complete exposition of the distribution, indications and acupoints of the Extraordinary Meridians does not appear until the Ming Dynasty (1368–1644 AD), in *A Study on the Eight Extraordinary Meridians* (*Qijing Bamai Kao*), written by Li Shizhen (1518–1593 AD) in 1578 AD[6].

Method of identification
As discussed in Chapter 1, it is likely that the pathways of the Regular Meridians were identified through the therapeutic application of heat (especially moxibustion) on the limbs, and the resulting awareness of the phenomenon of meridian transmission. However, this process would not have applied to the Extraordinary Meridians, which have no acupoints on the limbs. Rather, the identification of the Extraordinary Meridians was probably closely related to the practice of Taoist meditation techniques for the cultivation of *qi*, similar to today's *qigong* exercises. Both the Ren and Du Meridians originate in the lower abdomen at *dantian*, the Cinnabar Field or Sea of *Qi*. When the mind is successfully concentrated on this area, the flow of *qi* is activated within the Ren and Du Meridians, resulting in a sensation popularly known as the small cycle of *qi*. This amounts to stimulating meridian transmission through the Ren and Du Meridians by using internal mental concentration rather than external moxibustion. It is unlikely that these meditation techniques played a large part in the identification of the Regular Meridians, since only advanced adepts can psychically stimulate meridian transmission through the twelve Regular Meridians, the so-called large cycle of *qi*[7].

Distribution

The Regular Meridians follow a regular pattern of distribution, connecting internally with the *zangfu* organs and distributing externally to the limbs, trunk and head. The distribution of the eight Extraordinary Meridians is irregular. They have few connections with the internal *zangfu* organs, although several Extraordinary Meridians are related to the extraordinary organs. For instance, both the Ren and Du Meridians originate at the uterus, and the Du Meridian connects with the brain and spinal cord. Also, one Extraordinary Meridian usually connects with many Regular Meridians. For example, the Du Meridian connects with all of the Yang Meridians, and the Ren Meridian with all of the Yin Meridians.

Among the eight Extraordinary Meridians, only the Ren and Du Meridians are considered to take part in the cyclical flow of *qi* and blood throughout the body. (See Figure 2.2.)

Function

The Regular Meridians function to transport *qi* and blood, while the Extraordinary Meridians regulate the flow of *qi* and blood in the Regular Meridians. So if the Regular Meridians are compared to river courses, the Extraordinary Meridians are the lakes and seas. The two systems link up with each other to harmonize the flow of *qi* and blood throughout the body.

Acupoints

Each Regular Meridian has its own acupoints, but among the eight Extraordinary Meridians only the Ren and Du Meridians have their own acupoints. All other Extraordinary Meridians share acupoints with the Regular Meridians, with which they connect.

The fifteen collaterals

The fifteen collaterals, called *luo* or connectors in Chinese, are small branches of the meridians. Each of the Fourteen Meridians has one collateral, except for the Spleen Meridian, which has a second collateral called the major collateral of the Spleen Meridian. There is therefore a total of fifteen collaterals.

All collaterals derive from the meridians at specific acupoints, and are named after these acupoints. For example, the collateral of the Lung Meridian derives from LU7-Lieque, so it is called Lieque.

The twelve collaterals of the twelve Regular Meridians all originate below the elbow or knee. They are located superficially and connect with their interior–exterior related meridians. For example, the Lung Meridian (interior) is related to the Large Intestine Meridian (exterior). Therefore, the collateral of the Lung Meridian connects with the Large Intestine Meridian, while the collateral of the Large Intestine Meridian connects with the Lung Meridian.

The collaterals of the Ren and Du Meridians and the major collateral of the Spleen Meridian are distributed on the front, back and bilateral sides of the trunk respectively. The collateral of the Ren Meridian diverges from the Ren Meridian at the lower end of the sternum (RN15-Jiuwei), and then spreads over the abdomen. The collateral of the Du Meridian diverges from the Du Meridian at the sacral region (DU1-Changqiang), and then runs upward along the bilateral sides of the spine and spreads over the top of the head. The major collateral of the Spleen Meridian derives from the bilateral sides of the trunk at SP21-Dabao, and then spreads to the chest and hypochondriac regions.

The twelve collaterals of the twelve Regular Meridians strengthen the connection between the interior–exterior related meridians. The collaterals of the Ren and Du Meridians and the major collateral of the Spleen Meridian function to regulate the flow of *qi* and blood in the trunk.

Each collateral of the twelve Regular Meridians connects with two meridians, i.e. the Regular Meridian itself, and the Regular Meridian's interior–exterior related meridian. The points of origin of the collaterals, called *luo* (connecting) acupoints, can therefore be used to regulate disturbances of both the collateral's Regular Meridian itself, and the Regular Meridian's interior–exterior related meridian. For example, LU7-Lieque, the *luo* (connecting) acupoint of the collateral of the Lung Meridian, is effective for treating disorders of both the Lung Meridian and the Lung Meridian's interior–exterior related meridian, the Large Intestine Meridian. (See Chapter 3 for further discussion of the *luo* (connecting) acupoints.)

Applications of meridian theory

The system of meridians woven through the body is not only useful for visualizing the connections between the upper and lower and the internal and external parts of the body; it also provides an essential guide to the practice of traditional Chinese medicine, especially acupuncture. Meridian theory is the basis of all aspects of acupuncture, including diagnosis, pattern identification and selection of acupoints. The *Neijing* states[8]:

> The beginner starts by learning the twelve Regular Meridians, while the skillful practitioner need go no further. Those of mediocre skill think them simple, while adepts recognize their complexity.

Meridian diagnosis

The meridians connect internally with the *zangfu* organs, and are distributed externally over the surface of the entire body. Through the connections provided by the meridians, the upper part of the body is linked with the lower and the internal part with the external so that the body forms an organic whole. Pathologically, when meridians and their related *zangfu* organs or tissues are diseased, there will usually be manifestations on the meridians' external pathways. These may include visible changes, tenderness or nodes, decrease of skin electrical resistance, and changes in sensitivity to heat. These manifestations are instrumental in identifying which meridians are being affected and establishing a diagnosis. The process of meridian diagnosis utilizes the four primary methods of inspection, palpation, measurement of electrical resistance and measurement of sensitivity to heat.

Inspection
Meridian inspection consists of carefully checking for visible positive signs along the pathways of the meridians. Common visible positive signs and their indications include:

- Color changes, including red, white, and purple. A red color indicates acute and heat conditions; white indicates deficient and cold conditions; purple (usually with visible blood vessels) indicates pain or heat conditions.

☙ Eminences. These are usually localized. If an eminence is present, it should be palpated to determine whether it is soft or hard. Soft eminences (usually accompanied by severe tenderness) indicate acute conditions, while hard eminences indicate chronic conditions. Sometimes a soft eminence may appear only after pressure or massage of the meridians. This is also a valuable diagnostic sign.

☙ Pitting. This sign generally indicates chronic or deficient conditions. In many cases, the pitting occurs only after palpation or massage of the meridians, and takes a long time to recover.

☙ Pimples. Red pimples indicate heat or damp-heat conditions, while white pimples indicate cold or chronic conditions.

☙ Congestion of blood vessels. Visible red or purple blood vessels along the pathways of the meridians, especially on the popliteal fossa and elbow region, usually indicate heat or stagnant conditions.

☙ Desquamation. This usually indicates insufficiency of body fluid or skin problems.

☙ Others. There may also be instances of bleeding, sweating, or pigmented nevus along the meridians. These manifestations may indicate either pathological changes in the internal *zangfu* organs, or the meridians themselves. Some manifestations may be congenital, and should not be confused with pathological changes.

Precautions:

☙ Check the meridians under adequate light; do not stimulate the meridians before checking.

☙ Inspect the meridians from Root to Tip, i.e. from the limbs to the trunk and head. Pay particular attention to the Root segments on the limbs, especially around specific acupoints such as *yuan* (source), *xi* (cleft) and *he* (sea) acupoints.

☙ Visible changes are usually localized, and generally occur close to specific acupoints. It is relatively rare for changes to appear along sections or entire pathways of affected meridians.

☙ Distinguish the physiological from the pathological. Pigmented nevus along the meridians is usually congenital.

☙ Some visible changes, such as eminences and pitting, may occur only after stimulation of the meridians.

Palpation

Meridian palpation consists of palpating with steady pressure along the meridians with the ball of the thumb or an instrument with a rounded tip.

Main palpable signs include tenderness and hard nodes. Tenderness is the most commonly seen and most valuable sign in meridian diagnosis. Tenderness is a type of pain, but the patient is unaware of its presence until the tender area is pressed. Tenderness, like pain, is an alarm signaling that the body is in need of protection. The difference is that pain is a symptom, while tenderness is a sign. The patient is aware which part of the body is painful, but it is the practitioner's task to feel out the tender areas.

Tenderness may be a sign of a purely local problem – for example, in the case of tennis elbow, tenderness will be present in the affected region. However, more importantly, tenderness often indicates distal or general problems. When disease or disorder is present along the pathway of a meridian, or its internally connected organs are affected, there will usually be tenderness along the meridian, especially on its acupoints. For instance, in the case of lung problems there will usually be tenderness on the pathway of the Lung Meridian, especially LU1-Zhongfu, LU6-Kongzui, LU9-Taiyuan and LU10-Yuji.

The tender points that may occur along the pathways of meridians are not the same as the trigger points of Western medicine. Trigger points are abnormally tender locally, and pressing on them will trigger pain in their related areas. For instance, pressing trigger points on the trapezius, neck or temporal muscles may cause headache; pressing trigger points on the infraspinatus or supraspinatus muscles may cause shoulder pain. However, pressing tender points along the courses of the meridians will usually alleviate or even relieve the distal pain or other troubles immediately.

Tenderness can be classified into three grades:

1. Mild tenderness. The patient will declare pain only if asked whether or not there is pain, and there is no pain reaction such as flinching or crying out.
2. Moderate tenderness. The patient may declare pain without being asked, and there are pain reactions such as frowning or blinking.
3. Severe tenderness. The patient will usually declare stabbing pain, and may cry out and try to flinch away from the pressure.

Severe tender points are the most valuable diagnostic sign, as they indicate primarily affected meridians. The degree of tenderness depends mainly upon the nature and course of the condition. In general, tenderness will be severe in cases of acute or excessive conditions, but will be moderate or mild in cases of chronic or deficient conditions. Of course, there are also individual differences. Some people have a very high pain threshold, so it is almost impossible to locate tender points even when severe problems are present, whereas others may have such a low pain threshold that they report severe tenderness even though the condition is only moderate or mild.

Although in some cases the tender area may cover a section or even the entire pathway of the affected meridians, in most cases it is localized. The tender points generally coincide with the positions of classic acupoints. For instances, in cases of stomach problems there is usually tenderness at ST36-Zusanli; in cases of gallbladder disease there is usually tenderness at GB34-Yanglingquan.

'Hard nodes' refers to hard material, usually nodular, patchy or streaky in shape, located beneath the skin. They tend to occur near certain acupoints, especially the back *shu* (transport) and front *mu* (assembling) acupoints. Hard nodes generally indicate longstanding illness. For example, in cases of chronic gastritis or peptic ulcer, there may be nodes on the back *shu* (transport) acupoint of the stomach (UB21-Weishu).

Precautions:

- Palpate with even pressure and for the same length of time in order to avoid false positive or negative signs.
- Carefully observe the patient's reactions during palpation.
- Pay particular attention to acupoint regions, especially specific acupoints.
- Compare tender points with adjacent points several times. In most cases, the tender point can be precisely located.
- Tenderness is usually more severe on the affected side, so it is important to compare bilateral sides of a meridian in order to diagnose the location of the problem correctly.
- Look for pitting remaining after palpation. General speaking, deep whitish depressions with a long recovery time indicate deficient conditions, while shallow reddish depressions with a short recovery time indicate excessive conditions.
- Tenderness may be present in the absence of clinical symptoms, so this method is useful for early stage diagnosis.
- Changes in tenderness are valuable indications of prognosis. Tenderness will decrease as the condition improves, and finally disappear when a cure has been effected.

Measurement of electrical resistance

In 1950, the Japanese practitioner Nakatani Yoshio reported treating a case of severe nephritis. He found that many points on the surface of the body exhibited reduced electrical resistance. Surprisingly, the distribution of those points was identical with the pathway of the Kidney Meridian as recorded in the classic medical literature. Following further studies, he concluded that electrical resistance is lower along the pathways of the meridians, and that the meridians are good electrical conductors[9]. Further research revealed that in healthy people the electrical resistance of a meridian is similar on the bilateral sides of the body, indicating that the meridian is in balance. However, when illness occurs differences in electrical resistance appear, indicating that the meridian is out of balance. It is therefore possible to diagnose illness by measuring the electrical resistance of the meridians.

Measurement of electrical resistance has gained acceptance as a diagnostic method in many countries. The method involves measuring the electrical resistance of each Regular Meridian, usually on the *jing* (well) or *yuan* (source) acupoints. The meridian is considered out of balance if there is a significant difference in electrical resistance between its bilateral sides, or if the electrical resistance on the bilateral sides of the meridian is much lower than normal. Following diagnosis, acupoints of the affected meridians are selected and treated to restore balance.

Many factors may influence electrical resistance of the skin, especially pressure, duration of measurement, dampness of the skin, and general health. The following measures should therefore be taken to avoid false positive or negative results:

- The patient should rest for at least 10 minutes prior to measurement.
- The regions to be measured should not be washed or rubbed prior to measurement, in order to avoid false positive points, which may result from increased conduction due to congestion of blood. If the skin must be washed because it is seborrheic or dirty, there should be a 10-minute interval before measuring.
- The electrodes should be held with the correct force.
- The electrodes should not be held on one point for an extended period. Each acupoint should be measured within 2 seconds.
- Skin lesions such as injury, inflammation, pimples or scars will influence electrical conduction.
- Individual differences should be taken into account. Some people's electrical resistance is relatively high, making it difficult to detect positive points with this method, while that of others may be very low, resulting in easily occurring false positive points.

Measurement of sensitivity to heat

This diagnostic method was developed by Japanese practitioner Akabane Yukibei in 1950. While he was in bed with a severe case of tonsillitis, the second toe on his left foot was burned by accident. Although a large blister formed, he felt no pain in the burned area. He hypothesized that the insensitivity of the area, the approximate location of the *jing* (well) acupoint of the Stomach Meridian, was related to his tonsillitis, since the Stomach Meridian connects with the throat. Upon further investigation, he found a large sensitive area on the anterior region of his left thigh, located along the course of the Stomach Meridian. He then needled this area. Ten seconds after insertion of the needle he felt pain in the burned toe, and his tonsillitis quickly resolved.

Based upon this experience, the practitioner developed the following diagnostic method. One end of a slender stick of incense is ignited and tapped rhythmically on the *jing* (well) acupoint of each Regular Meridian, or held over the point, to determine how long it takes the patient to feel a burning sensation on the point. The *jing* (well) acupoints of diseased meridians will be relatively insensitive, and it will take longer for the patient to feel a burning sensation. This method is especially valuable in determining whether there is a major difference between the bilateral *jing* (well) acupoints of a meridian[10].

In clinical practice, the four methods of meridian diagnosis – inspection, palpation, measurement of electrical resistance and measurement of sensitivity to heat – can be used either singly or in combination. Meridian diagnosis allows accurate identification of the affected meridians, which is crucial for diagnosing disease and correctly selecting acupoints to treat the problem. Furthermore, it is helpful for assessing the progress of treatment, since positive signs along the meridians will decrease or disappear as the condition is alleviated or cured.

Pattern identification

Pattern identification is an essential component of traditional Chinese medicine, and provides the necessary foundation for effective treatment. To identify the pattern of a disorder, it is necessary to determine both the location and the properties of a condition at each stage of the disorder. Although the pattern is invisible, it is reflected in the ever-changing visible manifestations of the condition. Manifestations are appearance, while pattern is essence, and it is therefore possible to identify the invisible pattern by analyzing and synthesizing the visible manifestations. (See Appendix 5 for a complete discussion of pattern identification.)

According to traditional Chinese medicine, the human body consists of two systems, the *zangfu* organs and the meridians. Identifying the pattern of a disease involves determining which organs and meridians are being affected. The meridians, especially the twelve Regular Meridians, connect internally with the *zangfu* organs and are distributed externally over the surface of the body. The location of most diseases and disorders, either internal or external, can therefore be determined through the meridians.

Diseases are attributed to a meridian based on the meridian's pathway and connections. For example, the Large Intestine Meridian passes along the anterior border of the external side of the upper limb, and connects with the large intestine, lungs, throat, teeth and face. Therefore, disorders occurring along its course and connections, including tennis elbow, frozen shoulder, toothache, facial paralysis or spasm, trigeminal neuralgia, tonsillitis, upper respiratory tract infection and abdominal pain, are attributed to the Large Intestine Meridian.

Attribution of diseases to meridians has been a principal part of meridian theory since its inception. In the two oldest meridian texts from Mawangdui, discussions of each Regular Meridian include three elements – its pathway, its disorders, and methods of treating these disorders. The texts first describe the distribution of each meridian, then list the diseases and disorders that may occur along the course of the meridian, and finally discuss the application of moxibustion along the meridian to treat those problems. (See Appendices 2 and 3.)

Just as the pathway of each Regular Meridian can be divided into internal and external segments, so the diseases and disorders attributed to a Regular Meridian can also be classified into internal and external. Internal diseases refer to those that occur along the internal segment of a meridian (i.e. within the cavities of the trunk), while external problems are those that occur along the external segment of a meridian (i.e. on the limbs, surface of the trunk, neck and head).

There is generally no overlapping of the Regular Meridians on the limbs. Therefore, localized manifestations on the limbs are sufficient to identify the affected meridians. For instance, pain and numbness on the anterior border of the external side of the upper limb, on the pathway of the Large Intestine Meridian, can be attributed to this meridian; while pain on the anterior border of the external side of the lower limb, on the pathway of the Stomach Meridian, can be attributed to this meridian.

However, there is extensive overlapping and intersecting of the Regular Meridians on the trunk, head and internal organs. This means that one tissue or organ may be related to a number of meridians, and therefore localized manifestations in these areas are not sufficient to identify which meridians are being affected. Take the throat, for instance. The throat is related to the Lung, Large Intestine, Stomach, Liver, Gallbladder and Kidney Meridians. In a case of sore throat, therefore, additional manifestations must be taken into consideration in order to identify precisely the nature of the problem and which meridians or organs are being affected. If the condition is acute and accompanied by cough, fever and chills, it can be identified as invasion of the Lung Meridian by external pathogens; if it is acute but marked by a dry throat and bitter taste in the mouth, and accompanied by restlessness, irritability and headache, it can be identified as flaming upward of liver fire; while if the condition is chronic and marked by a dry throat and mild pain accompanied by afternoon fever, night sweating, restlessness and the sensation of heat in the palms and soles, it will be identified as yin deficiency of the lung and kidney.

Clinical advantages of meridian theory over *zangfu* theory

Meridian theory has the following major advantages over *zangfu* theory in the clinical practice of acupuncture:

1. Because the meridians are distributed over the entire body, they can be used to identify affected meridians in cases that are not addressed by *zangfu* theory. For instance, according to *zangfu* theory there is no internal organ associated with the neck. However, it is very easy to identify the source of problems of the neck using meridian theory. Disorders on the front of the neck, such as problems of the thyroid gland, are attributed to the Stomach and Large Intestine Meridians, which pass through this area; problems on the bilateral sides of the neck, such as mumps and stiff neck, are attributed to the Gallbladder and San Jiao Meridians, which pass through this area; conditions of the back of the neck, such as stiff neck and cervical spondylopathy, are attributed to the Urinary Bladder and Du Meridians, which pass through this area.

2. Better results can be obtained by treating acupoints of the meridian directly related to the problem area, rather than acupoints of the meridian of the *zangfu* organ related to the problem area. Take the ears, for instance. The meridians closely connecting with the ears are the San Jiao (called the Ear Meridian in the *Classic of Moxibustion with Eleven Yin-Yang Meridians*), Gallbladder and Small Intestine Meridians. According to *zangfu* theory, the kidneys open into the ears. However, according to meridian theory there is no direct connection between the kidneys and ears. Accordingly, it is preferable to treat diseases of the ear with acupoints of the San Jiao, Gall Bladder and Small Intestine Meridians, which have a direct connection with the ears, rather than with acupoints of the Kidney Meridian, the meridian of the ears' related *zangfu* organ. (See Table 2.4.)

In conclusion, meridian theory is essential to the practice of acupuncture. Once a problem has been attributed to a meridian, acupoints of the affected meridians can be selected for effective treatment.

Table 2.4
Treatment of ear problems with Kidney Meridian acupoints versus San Jiao, Gallbladder and Small Intestine Meridian acupoints (based on the *Classic of Bright Halls*, the oldest monograph on acupoints)

Meridians	*Total number of acupoints below elbows and knees*	*Number of acupoints below elbows and knees indicated for ear problems*	*Percentage of total acupoints below elbows and knees indicated for ear problems*
San Jiao Meridian	10	5	50
Small Intestine Meridian	8	5	62.5
Gallbladder Meridian	11	2	18.2
Kidney Meridian	10	0	0

Disorders of the Fourteen Meridians

Lung Meridian of Hand Taiyin

- *Internal disorders.* The Lung Meridian connects internally with the lung, large intestine, trachea and cardia. Its internal disorders therefore include: cough, asthma, shortness of breath and pain or feeling of fullness in the chest; hemoptysis; vomiting; hiccups; acute diarrhea; abdominal pain.
- *External disorders.* The Lung Meridian connects externally with the throat and runs along the supraclavicular fossa and the anterior border of the medial aspect of the upper limb. Its external disorders therefore include: swelling and pain of the throat; pain in the supraclavicular fossa; shoulder pain aggravated by abduction; pain, numbness and skin problems along its pathway on the upper limb.

Large Intestine Meridian of Hand Yangming

- *Internal disorders.* The Large Intestine Meridian connects internally with the large intestine and lung. Its internal disorders therefore include: abdominal pain; diarrhea; constipation; cough and pain in the chest.
- *External disorders.* The Large Intestine Meridian runs externally along the anterior border of the lateral aspect of the upper limb, ascends along the lateral side of the neck, and connects with the teeth (especially the lower teeth), mouth, face and nose. Its Divergent Meridian connects with the throat. Its external disorders therefore include: pain, numbness and skin problems along its pathway on the upper limb; shoulder pain; swelling of the neck; swelling and pain of the teeth, especially the lower teeth; deviation of the mouth, facial pain or spasm; nasal discharge or obstruction; hyposmia; swelling and pain of the throat.

Stomach Meridian of Foot Yangming

- *Internal disorders.* The Stomach Meridian connects internally with the stomach and spleen; its Divergent Meridian connects with the heart. Its internal problems include: stomachache; distension in the upper abdomen; poor appetite or frequent hunger; anorexia; vomiting; hiccups; insomnia; manic or depressive mental disorders; epilepsy.

☯ *External disorders*. The Stomach Meridian is distributed externally over the face, forehead, front of trunk, and along the anterior border of the lateral side of the lower limb; it connects with the nose, eyes, lips, thyroid gland and breasts. Its external disorders include: facial pain, paralysis or spasm; nasal discharge, obstruction or bleeding; pain of the eyeball; swelling and redness of the eyes; blurred vision; swelling and pain of the lips; headache, especially in the frontal area; goiter; swelling and pain of the breasts; lumps in the breasts; pain, numbness or other problems along its course on the lower limb.

Spleen Meridian of Foot Taiyin

☯ *Internal disorders*. The Spleen Meridian connects internally with the spleen, stomach, heart and esophagus. Its internal disorders therefore include: stomachache; distension in the epigastric region; poor appetite and anorexia; vomiting; diarrhea; constipation; abdominal pain; menstrual disorders; edema; insomnia; manic or depressive disorders; pain of the esophagus or difficulty in swallowing.

☯ *External disorders*. The Spleen Meridian runs externally along the anterior border of the medial side of the lower limb, and connects with the throat and root of the tongue. Its external disorders therefore include: pain, numbness or other problems along its course on the lower limb; sensation of foreign object in the throat; spasm or paralysis of the tongue; salivation; lower abdominal pain.

Heart Meridian of Hand Shaoyin

☯ *Internal disorders*. The Heart Meridian connects internally with the heart, small intestine and lungs. Its internal disorders therefore include: cardiac pain and palpitations; insomnia; manic or depressive disorders; profuse or suppressed sweating; pain or feeling of fullness in the chest; shortness of breath; thirst.

☯ *External disorders*. The Heart Meridian runs externally along the posterior border of the medial side of the upper limb and connects with the throat and eyes; its collateral connects with the root of tongue. Its external problems therefore include: pain, numbness or other problems along its pathway on the upper limb; dry throat; yellow eyes; rigidity of the tongue.

Small Intestine Meridian of Hand Taiyang

☯ *Internal disorders*. The Small Intestine Meridian connects internally with the small intestine, heart, esophagus and stomach. Its internal disorders therefore include: insufficient lactation; pain of the esophagus; stomachache.

☯ *External disorders*. The Small Intestine Meridian runs externally over the posterior border of the lateral side of the upper limb, curves around the scapular region, and ascends along the lateral side of the neck; it connects with the ears, nose and eyes. Its external problems therefore include: pain, numbness or other problems along its course on the upper limb; pain and motor impairment of the shoulder; stiff neck; tinnitus; deafness; pain or discharge from the ears; nasal discharge or obstruction; yellow eyes; blurred vision.

Urinary Bladder Meridian of Foot Taiyang

☙ *Internal disorders.* The Urinary Bladder Meridian connects internally with the urinary bladder, kidneys and brain; its Divergent Meridian connects with the heart. Its internal disorders therefore include: difficult or frequent urination; urinary incontinence; nocturnal enuresis; epilepsy; manic or depressive mental disorders.

☙ *External disorders.* The Urinary Bladder Meridian is distributed externally on the areas between the eyebrows, the top of the head, occipital region, back of the neck, trunk and lower limb; it connects with the eyes. Its Divergent Meridian connects with the anus. Its external disorders therefore include: pain in the supraorbital region; headache, especially in the occipital region; stiff neck; backache; pain, numbness, coldness or other problems along its course on the lower limb; myopia; yellow eyes; lacrimation induced by wind; hemorrhoids; prolapse of the anus.

Kidney Meridian of Foot Shaoyin

☙ *Internal disorders.* The Kidney Meridian connects internally with the kidneys, urinary bladder, liver, lungs and heart. Its internal disorders therefore include: urinary incontinence; nocturnal enuresis; impotence; involuntary seminal emission; anxiety; dizziness; tinnitus; blurred vision; poor memory; jaundice; diarrhea; shortness of breath; difficulty in inhaling; palpitations; restlessness; insomnia.

☙ *External disorders.* The Kidney Meridian runs externally through the heel and along the posterior border of the medial side of the lower limb; it connects with the spinal column, throat and root of the tongue. Its external disorders therefore include: pain, numbness, coldness or other problems along its course on the lower limb; heel pain; lower back pain; dry throat; swelling and pain of the throat; dry tongue; thirst; salty taste in the mouth.

Pericardium Meridian of Hand Jueyin

☙ *Internal disorders.* The Pericardium Meridian connects internally with the pericardium and San Jiao. Its internal disorders therefore include: pain or fullness in the chest; palpitations; depression; restlessness; manic or depressive disorders; nausea; vomiting; hiccups; gastric pain; distension in the upper abdomen.

☙ *External disorders.* The Pericardium Meridian is distributed externally over the hypochondriac region and the middle section of the medial aspect of the upper limb. Its external disorders therefore include: pain, numbness, coldness or other problems along its course on the upper limb; pain in the hypochondriac region.

San Jiao Meridian of Hand Shaoyang

☙ *Internal disorders.* The San Jiao Meridian connects internally with the San Jiao and pericardium. Its internal disorders therefore include: pain in the chest; hiccups; constipation; nocturnal enuresis.

☙ *External disorders.* The San Jiao Meridian runs externally along the middle section of the external side of the upper limb, ascends along the lateral side of the neck, curves around the root of the ear, and connects with the ears and the outer canthus of the eye. Its external disorders therefore include: pain, numbness, coldness or other problems along its course on the upper limb; shoulder pain; stiff neck; pain behind the ears; pain or discharge from the ears; tinnitus; loss of hearing; redness and swelling of the eyes.

Gallbladder Meridian of Foot Shaoyang

☯ *Internal disorders*. The Gall Bladder Meridian connects internally with the gallbladder and liver; its Divergent Meridian connects with the heart. Its internal disorders therefore include: pain and distension in the hypochondriac region; aversion to fatty foods; poor appetite; frequent sighing; depression, anxiety and indecision; heart pains; palpitations; mental disorders.

☯ *External disorders*. The Gall Bladder Meridian descends externally along the lateral side of the body from head to foot and connects with the ears and face; its Divergent Meridian connects with the throat and the tissues (primarily nerves and blood vessels) that link the eyeball and brain. Its external disorders therefore include: headache, especially in the temporal region; pain or discharge from the ears; tinnitus; sudden loss of hearing; swelling and pain of the eyes; poor vision; lacrimation induced by wind; myopia; distension and pain of the eyeball; dusty facial complexion; facial pain, paralysis, spasm or itching; bitter taste in the mouth; sensation of foreign object in the throat; stiff neck; shoulder pain; pain or skin diseases in the hypochondriac region; hip pain; pain, numbness, coldness or other problems along its course on the lower limb.

Liver Meridian of Foot Jueyin

☯ *Internal disorders*. The Liver Meridian connects internally with the liver, gallbladder, lungs and stomach. Its internal disorders therefore include: pain and distension in the hypochondriac region; frequent sighing; depression, restlessness and irritability; depressive or manic mental disorders; hysteria; cough; asthma; feeling of fullness in the chest; gastric pain; nausea; vomiting; hiccups; anorexia; diarrhea.

☯ *External disorders*. The Liver Meridian runs externally along the middle section of the medial side of the lower limb, passes the inguinal groove, connects with the throat and eyes, spreads over the inside of the cheek and lips, and ends at the top of the head. There is a close relation between the Liver Meridian and the external genitals; its collateral meridian, Divergent Meridian and muscle region, as well as the main course, all directly connect with this region. Its external disorders therefore include: pain, numbness, coldness or other problems along its course on the lower limb; inguinal hernia; pain, swelling or itching in the external genital region; impotence; seminal emission; priapism; prolapse of the uterus; dysmenorrhea, irregular menstruation, leukorrhagia; dry throat; sensation of foreign object in the throat; pain and distension of the eyeballs; blurred vision; myopia.

Du Meridian

☯ *Internal disorders*. The Du Meridian enters the skull and connects with the brain, the extraordinary organ that dominates mental activities. Its internal disorders therefore include: various mental disorders, such as poor memory; dizziness; insomnia; depression; mania; loss of consciousness; epilepsy.

☯ *External disorders*. The Du Meridian runs along the midline of the back. Its external disorders therefore include: acute lumbar sprain; lumbar muscle strain; stiff neck; pain of the spinal column.

The Du Meridian is the Sea of all Yang Meridians, functioning both to clear heat and to warm the body as needed. It is therefore associated with disorders including: febrile diseases; malaria; carbuncles; cellulitis; boils; aversion to cold; retention of urine; incontinence of urine; nocturnal enuresis; infertility.

Ren Meridian

The Ren Meridian originates from the uterus in the female, and *jinggong*, the Palace of Essence, in the male, descending to distribute through the external genital region. It is therefore associated with gynecological disorders and disorders of the external genitals, including: pain, distension or itching in the external genital region; swelling and pain of the testicles; prolapse of the uterus; dysmenorrhea; irregular menstruation; leukorrhagia; pain or lumps in the lower abdomen; infertility.

The Ren Meridian passes through the Middle Jiao, the source of phlegm. Accumulation of turbid phlegm will disturb the heart and lead to mental problems, so the Ren Meridian is associated with disorders including mania, depression and hysteria.

The Ren Meridian passes through the San Jiao. It is therefore associated with disorders of the Lower Jiao including retention of urine; incontinence and nocturnal enuresis; disorders of the Middle Jiao including pain and distension in the upper abdomen, anorexia, vomiting and hiccups; and disorders of the Upper Jiao including cough, asthma, shortness of breath, pain or feeling of fullness in the chest.

Selection of acupoints

The acupoints of the Fourteen Meridians are specific sites located along the pathways of these meridians. Each of the Fourteen Meridians is associated with various diseases and disorders. One of the basic principles of acupuncture and meridian theory is to treat a disorder with acupoints located on the meridian associated with the disorder. The *Classic of Moxibustion with Eleven Yin-Yang Meridians* and Chapter 10 of the *Lingshu* describe the distribution of each meridian, and list two types of associated disorders. The first group consists of disorders resulting from disturbance of the meridian, while the second consists of disorders indicated for treatment using the meridian. The second group of disorders consists of those located primarily along the course of the meridian or its connections. Both types of disorders are treated using acupoints located on the associated meridian. (See Appendices 3 and 4.)

Although the therapeutic applications of the acupoints are numerous and complex, they can be easily mastered by understanding the pathways and connections of each meridian, and the meridians' associated disorders. The meridians, rather than the acupoints, are the primary means for determining treatment. Yang Jizhou (1522–1619 AD), an eminent practitioner of the Ming dynasty (1368–1644 AD), suggests in the *Compendium of Acupuncture and Moxibustion*: 'Better to forego the acupoints than the meridians'[11].

Case histories

The value of selecting acupoints according to meridian theory is particularly apparent when using acupoints of the twelve Regular Meridians located below the elbow and knee, and points of the Du and Ren Meridians. Most of these points can be used to treat not only local conditions, but also distal disorders located along the course of the meridian quite far away from the points. A typical case is offered for each of the Fourteen Meridians in order to clarify this principle.

Cough (Lung Meridian)
I was once sick with a case of acute bronchitis that had lasted for over a month. There was profuse dilute sputum, sometimes white and sometimes yellow. I had tried various

medications, both modern and traditional, but with no improvement. One day as I was pressing along the left Lung Meridian between the wrist and elbow, I found there was severe tenderness in the region of LU6-Kongzui. When I rolled up my sleeve, I was surprised to discover a reddened eminence about 1.5 cm in diameter at the site of the acupoint. I punctured the acupoint with a fine needle, and the soreness and distension in my left forearm was so strong that I could not move my arm. This was the first time I had ever experienced such a strong needling sensation. Following the needling I felt much better, and coughed up some sputum. The next day I was completely recovered. There was only moderate tenderness on the acupoint, and no strong needling sensation occurred when I needled it again.

Chronic diarrhea (Large Intestine Meridian)

A 40-year-old woman had suffered from chronic diarrhea for many years. The condition was diagnosed as chronic colitis in modern medical terms, but neither modern nor Chinese herbal medicine had yielded any improvement. Manifestations included frequent diarrhea (four to seven times a day), occasional bloody stool, abdominal pain and distension, and poor appetite. Colonoscopy revealed reddened and swollen intestinal mucosa and the presence of several superficial ulcers. The condition was identified as accumulation of damp heat in the large intestine. Bilateral LI1-Shangyang, the *jing* (well) points of the Large Intestine Meridian, were pricked with a three-edged needle to let 0.5–1.0 ml blood on each acupoint, once every other day. Five treatments constituted one course. There was great improvement in all symptoms after one course of treatment. No discomfort remained after two courses of treatment, and the patient exhibited good appetite and renewed vigor. The practitioner reported using this method to treat many cases of chronic colitis and functional disturbance following colon surgery during his 40 years' practice[12].

Headache (Stomach Meridian)

A 20-year-old man complained of soreness and spasm of the legs. The problem had started one morning after he was caught out in the rain. Bilateral ST41-Jiexi were selected as local acupoints to activate the flow of *qi* and blood and relieve pain. During manipulation of the needles, the patient felt a needling sensation ascending along the lower limbs and terminating at the head. Ten minutes later the local pain disappeared and he could walk freely. What was more surprising was that his longstanding headache was also relieved[13].

Tongue retraction (Spleen Meridian)

An old man complained of tongue retraction. The problem had appeared 3 days previously, simultaneous with diarrhea. Both medicine and acupuncture (acupoints including DU16-Fengfu and RN23-Lianquan) had been given but with no improvement. As well as tongue retraction, additional manifestations included loose stool, bland taste in the mouth, thin whitish tongue coating and soggy pulse. Because the Spleen Meridian connects with the root of the tongue and spreads over the inferior surface of the tongue, deficient spleen *qi* can result in insufficient fluid to nourish the tongue, and resulting stiffness of the tongue. The condition was identified as deficiency of spleen *qi*. SP3-Taibai and ST36-Zusanli, the *yuan* (source) acupoint of the Spleen Meridian and *he* (sea) acupoint of the Stomach Meridian were needled using the reinforcing method in combination with moxibustion. Local points Ex-Jinjin and Ex-Yuye were also punctured. The next day the patient could extend his tongue and the stool had solidified. One more treatment resulted in a cure[14].

Night sweating (Heart Meridian)
A 28-year-old woman complained of night sweating. The condition had been diagnosed as pulmonary tuberculosis. Antituberculotic and antiperspirant medication had been given, but with no improvement in the sweating. Perspiration is the humor of the heart, so sweating can occur if the heart *qi* is insufficient to maintain its humor within the body. Bilateral HT6-Yinxi, the *xi* (cleft) acupoints of the Heart Meridian, were stimulated with three medium-sized cones of moxa. The next morning the patient reported a noticeable reduction in sweating that night. Following three additional treatments, the night sweating stopped completely. The practitioner reported curing eight cases of night sweating with this method[15].

Tympanitis (Small Intestine Meridian)
The patient exhibited a discharge of pus from the right ear and severe pain around the auricle. The pain on the front of the auricle disappeared after puncturing right SI3-Houxi using the reducing method, and the pain on the back of the auricle disappeared after puncturing right SJ3-Zhongzhu using the reducing method. The Small Intestine Meridian enters the ear from the anterior region of the auricle, and the San Jiao Meridian enters the ear from the posterior region, so acupoints of these two meridians can effectively relieve pain in their corresponding regions[16].

Occipital pain (Urinary Bladder Meridian)
A 46-year-old woman had suffered from intermittent headache, primarily in the occipital region, for 5 years. She had been treated with various methods but with no improvement. The condition had recently become worse. Additional manifestations included dizziness and poor appetite, deep and thready pulse, and white tongue coating. Since the pain was located along the course of the Urinary Bladder Meridian, UB67-Zhiyin was punctured using the even method to dredge the meridian and relieve pain. The patient was cured with a total of four treatments[17].

Asthma (Kidney Meridian)
A 62-year-old woman had been living with asthma for over 20 years. The condition became worse every spring and summer. She had tried many kinds of modern and herbal medicines, but with no radical cure. She had difficulty breathing, especially inhaling, aggravated by exertion. Her tongue was pale with a whitish greasy coating, and the pulse was deep and slightly slippery. The condition was identified as deficiency of the kidney *qi*, resulting in failure to absorb *qi*. Bilateral KI3-Taixi, the *shu* (stream) and *yuan* (source) acupoint of the Kidney Meridian, were punctured using the reinforcing method to supplement the kidney *qi*. She was cured with a total of twenty treatments, and there was no relapse over a 3-year follow-up[18].

Hysteria (Pericardium Meridian)
A 32-year-old woman was experiencing hysteria. The problem had manifested 1 month previously, with no specific precipitating factor. Manifestations included pain in the chest, restlessness, intermittent laughing and crying, anxiety, and constipation. The condition was aggravated at night, and sometimes she could not sleep all night. Her tongue tip was reddened with a whitish greasy coating, and the pulse was wiry and slippery. The condition was identified as hysteria due to the combination of stagnant liver *qi* and accumulated phlegm, resulting in disturbance of the heart. Bilateral PC6-Neiguan, the *luo* (connecting) acupoint of the Pericardium Meridian and the *hui* (confluence) acupoint of the Yinwei Meridian, were needled using the even method to quicken the flow of *qi*, widen the chest,

loosen phlegm and tranquillize the mind, treating both the Root and Tip of the problem. As soon as the needles were inserted at a slight upward slant, the patient experienced a needling sensation in the chest and reported feeling calm and comfortable. Du26-Renzhong was needled at the same time for tranquillization. The patient felt fine after retaining the needles for half-an-hour. There was no relapse over a 2-year follow-up[19].

Hearing loss (San Jiao Meridian)

A 35-year-old man complained of hearing loss. He had experienced sudden hearing loss in his right ear accompanied by dizziness and nausea 1 week previously, with no definite cause. The following day the hearing in his left ear was also impaired. The edges of his tongue were purple, and it had a thin yellow coating. The pulse was deep and wiry. The condition was identified as nervous deafness due to upward flaring of San Jiao fire. Bilateral SJ3-Zhongzhu were punctured using the reducing method to clear fire and sharpen the ears. There was improvement in his hearing after the first treatment, and he was cured with a total of five treatments[20].

Headache (Gallbladder Meridian)

An old man reported having had headaches for over 10 years. He had been treated with many methods but with no improvement. GB39-Xuanzhong was punctured on the affected side. Upon insertion of the needle, the patient reported a strong needling sensation, similar to electric shock, radiating from the acupoint to his head, and immediate alleviation of the pain. Three minutes after insertion of the needle, the pain disappeared completely. He was cured with just one treatment and there was no relapse over a 10-year follow-up[21].

Dysmenorrhea and vertex pain (Liver Meridian)

A 26-year-old woman reported having dysmenorrhea for 10 years. She took painkillers every month, but this time they hadn't been effective. In addition to pain in the lower abdomen, there was also severe pain on the vertex. The liver functions to regulate the flow of *qi* and blood, and the Liver Meridian ascends to the vertex. The condition was identified as stagnation of the liver *qi*. Bilateral LR3-Taichong, which are both the *shu* (stream) and *yuan* (source) acupoints of the Liver Meridian, were needled to quicken the flow of *qi* and blood and relieve pain. The pain in the lower abdomen and on the vertex was relieved after the first treatment. There was no pain over several months follow-up. The practitioner has treated many such cases, with one treatment sufficient for the majority[22].

Low tolerance for cold (Du Meridian)

An adult man complained of always feeling cold, even when covered with thick cotton-wadded quilts during the summer. Additional manifestations included dizziness, lassitude, bright white facial complexion, sensation of cold in the extremities, dry body with no sweating, and occasional feelings of cold on the back. The condition was identified as yang deficiency. DU14-Dazhui, located at the intersection of the Du Meridian and all Yang Meridians, was heated with moxa to invigorate yang *qi*. Following application of three medium-sized cones of moxa, there was slight sweating over his entire body, and his hands and feet warmed up to a normal temperature. The condition was cured with only one treatment[23].

Headache (Ren Meridian)

A 50-year-old woman reported having headaches for 10 years, marked by pain in the front of the head and a heavy, swathed feeling. Oral administration of both modern and Chinese herbal medicines had resulted in some improvement, but the condition had worsened over the last several years. Additional symptoms included blurred vision, a feeling of fullness in the chest and epigastric region, nausea, vomiting of phlegm, poor appetite, abdominal distension after eating, lassitude, emaciation and loose stool. Her tongue was pale with a greasy coating, and the pulse was wiry and slippery. The condition was identified as headache due to turbid phlegm in the Middle Jiao obstructing the ascent of clear *qi* to nourish the brain. RN12-Zhongwan, which is both the front *mu* (assembly) acupoint of the stomach and the *hui* (influential) acupoint of the six *fu* organs, was needled using the reducing method to loosen phlegm and allow ascent of clear *qi*. The pain was relieved after just one treatment and there was no relapse during a 2-year follow-up. In this case, the headache was the Tip and the turbid phlegm in the Middle Jiao was the Root. Treating the headache would therefore not have been effective, but severing its Root yielded tangible results. The practitioner reported successfully treating many cases of frontal headache using this method, with minimal treatments necessary[24].

Notes and References

1. *Lingshu*, 10:30.
2. *Ibid*, 38:79.
3. Dou Hanqing (*c*. 1196–1280 AD), *Lyrics of Standard Profundities (Biao You Fu* 标幽赋). Quoted in Yang Jizhou, *Compendium of Acupuncture and Moxibustion (Zhenjiu Dacheng* 针灸大成) (1601 AD). Beijing: People's Health Press, 1963, p. 48. The *Compendium of Acupuncture and Moxibustion* was compiled by Yang Jizhou (*c*. 1522–1619 AD) in 1601 AD. This work was translated into Latin by Portuguese, French, Dutch and Danish missionaries, traders and physicians travelling and working in China and Japan from the seventeenth to the nineteenth centuries, and was the primary source of information concerning acupuncture in Europe during this time.
4. *Lingshu*, 5:16.
5. For details, see Cheng Xinnong *et al.*, *Chinese Acupuncture and Moxibustion*. Beijing: Foreign Languages Press, 1987.
6. Li Shizhen (1518–1593 AD) published an extensive study on the distribution and functions of the Extraordinary Meridians in 1578 AD, entitled *A Study on the Eight Extraordinary Meridians (Qijing Bamai Kao* 奇经八脉考). He is also famous for compiling the *Compendium of Materia Medica (Bencao Gangmu* 本草纲目) in 1590 AD.
7. Wang Buxiong *et al.*, *Developmental History of Chinese Qigong (Zhongguo Qigong Xueshu Fazhanshi* 中国气功学术发展史). Changshan: Hunan Science and Technology Publishing House, 1989, p. 434.
8. *Lingshu*, 11:39.
9. Wang Benxian, *Foreign Research on the Meridians*, p. 390.
10. *Ibid.*, p. 385.
11. Yang Yizhou, *Compendium of Acupuncture and Moxibustion*, p. 49.
12. Lu Jingshan *et al.*, *A Collection of Treatments Using One Acupoint (Danxue Zhibing Xuancui* 单穴治病选粹). Beijing: People's Health Press, 1993, p. 22.
13. Huang Jiaocheng, *Journal of Traditional Chinese Medicine (Zhongyi Zazhi* 中医杂志), 1957, 8:437.
14. Qin Liangpu, *Shanghai Journal of Acupuncture and Moxibustion (Shanghai Zhenjiu Zazhi* 上海针灸杂志), 1993, 12(1):38.
15. Liu Jianmin, *Zhejiang Journal of Traditional Chinese Medicine (Zhejiang Zhongyi Zazhi* 浙江中医杂志, 1957, 10:14.
16. Li Shizhen, *Discussion on the Utilization of Commonly Used Acupuncture Points (Changyong Shuxue Linchuang Fahui* 常用腧穴临床发挥). Beijing: People's Health Press, 1985, p. 354.
17. He Puren, *Relief of Pain with Acupuncture (Zhenjiu Zhitong* 针灸治痛). Beijing: Scientific and Technical Documents Publishing House, 1995, p. 29.

18. Lu Jingshan *et al.*, *A Collection of Treatments Using One Acupoint*, p. 191.
19. Yang Meiliang, *Zhejiang Journal of Traditional Chinese Medicine* (*Zhejiang Zhongyi Zazhi* 浙江中医杂志), 1980, 8:368.
20. He Puren, *Acupuncture Needling Methods* (*Zhenju Zhenfa* 针具针法). Beijing: Scientific and Technical Documents Publishing House, 1989, p. 190.
21. Yuan Boyuan, *Shanghai Journal of Acupuncture and Moxibustion*, 1987, 1:45.
22. Lu Jingshan *et al.*, *A Collection of Treatments Using One Acupoint*, p. 278.
23. Yu Maoji, *Discussion on the Properties of DU14-Dazhui*. Unpublished Conference Material, 1994.
24. He Puren, *Relief of Pain with Acupuncture*, p. 39.

Chapter 3
Acupoints – the terminals of the network

'All three hundred and sixty-five *qixue* (caves of *qi*) are areas through which the needles enter the body.'
Suwen

The acupoints are sites on the skin, often located in small depressions, where the *qi* and blood flowing through the meridians converge. The modern Chinese medical term for acupoint, *shuxue* (transportation cave), reflects this phenomenon, as do the classical terms *qixue* (cave of *qi*), *qihui* (confluence of *qi*) and *qifu* (mansion of *qi*) used in the *Neijing*. Acupoints are considered to be the 'gates' of the meridians, the points where the *qi* and blood come closest to the surface and are most accessible. If the interconnected meridians resemble a network, the acupoints are their terminals. Penetration of needles into the body through these gates can remove obstructions in the meridians and quicken the circulation of *qi* and blood. This chapter will discuss the discovery and classification of the acupoints, their effects, specific acupoints, and acupoint diagnosis.

Discovery of the acupoints

The meridians, acupoints and acupuncture are closely related and function together. Because of their deep interconnection, they have historically often been considered to be one system. However, it has been demonstrated in the previous chapters that the identification of the meridians actually preceded the invention of acupuncture. The invention of acupuncture would not have been possible without the prior identification of the meridians by the Chinese ancestors, and their holistic realization that they could stimulate the flow of *qi* through the meridians by needling specific points, just as they channeled the flow of water through the Earth's river courses by dredging certain areas.

Historical references

Now we arrive at the question of how the acupoints, the gateways to the body's *qi*, were discovered. First, let us review historical references to the meridians, acupuncture and the acupoints, in chronological order.

Ancient Medical Relics of Mawangdui (c. prior to 168 BC)
The *Ancient Medical Relics of Mawangdui*, which contain the two oldest known texts concerning the meridians, make no mention of needling or acupoints. These documents

discuss the application of moxibustion to the general meridians and diseased or very large areas, rather than to specific points.

Historical Records (c. 104–91 BC)
The first mention of needling is found in the *Historical Records*, in the biography of Cang Gong (*c.* 215–140 BC). Cang Gong, the first recorded practitioner of traditional Chinese medicine, lived during the early part of the Western Han Dynasty (206 BC–24 AD) at the time of the birth of acupuncture. In four of the cases mentioned in the biography, Cang Gong applied moxibustion or needling to the general meridians and adjoining areas. However, no specific acupoints were mentioned in his treatments. The places he needled, referred to as *suo* (areas), were without names or precise locations. (See Table 3.1.)

Table 3.1
Cang Gong's four moxibustion and needling cases
(based on Chapter 105 of *Historical Records*, pp. 486–94)

Disease	Therapy	Areas	Repetitions
Difficulty in urination, yellow urine, swelling of lower abdomen	Moxibustion	One *suo* (area) on each side of Foot Jueyin Meridian	One treatment
Hot sensation in feet, restlessness	Needling	Three *suo* (areas) on each side of the sole	One treatment
Tooth decay	Moxibustion	Left Hand Yangming Meridian	One treatment
Headache, fever, restlessness	Needling	Three *suo* (areas) on each side of Foot Yangming Meridian	One treatment

Neijing (c. 104–32 BC)
The *Neijing* is the oldest extant document to mention specific acupoints. Four chapters include discussions of acupoints[1]. The *Neijing* states that there are 365 acupoints, corresponding to the 365 days of the year, although only 160 are mentioned by name[2]. The following points indicate that the *Neijing*, the seminal work of traditional Chinese medicine, was compiled at the beginning of the transition from stimulation of the general meridians to stimulation of specific acupoints.

First, the *Neijing*, like the *Ancient Medical Relics of Mawangdui*, generally calls for treatment of the general meridians rather than specific points. Examples include[3–5]:

In cases of retention of urine, puncture the Foot Shaoyin and Foot Taiyang Meridians, and the sacral region with long needles.

In cases of dry throat or heat and sticky sensation in the mouth, select the Foot Shaoyin Meridian; in cases of sore throat, select the Foot Yangming Meridian if the patient cannot speak, but select the Hand Yangming Meridian if the patient can speak.

In cases of toothache, select the Foot Yangming Meridian if the patient prefers cold drinks, but select the Hand Yangming Meridian if the patient shows an aversion to cold drinks.

In cases of deafness, select the Foot Shaoyang Meridian if there is no pain, but select the Hand Shaoyang Meridian if there is pain.

Second, even when the *Neijing* mentions specific acupoints it calls for needling of the general anatomical regions where they are located rather than the points themselves. For instance[6–9]:

> In cases of wind type tetany, first needle the Foot Taiyang Meridian and its collateral on the popliteal fossa [approximate location of UB40-Weizhong] to cause bleeding. Combine with Sanli [approximate location of ST36-Zusanli] if there is interior cold.

> In cases of retention of urine, needle the Yinqiao Meridian and the area on the top of the big toe [approximate location of LR1-Dadun] to cause bleeding.

> In cases of deafness, select the regions at the meeting of the nail and flesh of the fourth finger and toe [approximate location of SJ1-Guanchong and GB44-Zuqiaoyin]. First needle the finger and then the toe.

> In cases of blurred vision and dizziness, select the area below the outer side of the ankle joint [approximate location of UB62-Shenmai].

> In cases of flaccidity, cold limbs, and restlessness, needle the area 2 *cun* above the web between the big and second toes [approximate location of LR3-Taichong].

> In cases of Foot Yangming type malaria, needle the dorsal section of the Foot Yangming Meridian [approximate location of ST42-Chongyang].

The *Neijing* indicates that the acupoints on the limbs, especially those below the elbows and knees, were the first to be discovered. Among the 160 acupoints recorded in the *Neijing*, eighty-two are located below the elbows and knees. These eighty-two original points account for 71 per cent of the 114 acupoints below the elbows and knees in use today. The names and locations of these points have not changed since they were first recorded. These acupoints are discussed in detail in the *Lingshu* section of the *Neijing*, while the more recent *Suwen* section concentrates on acupoints on the trunk and head, only mentioning those on the limbs in passing[10]. It can therefore be inferred that stimulation, either moxibustion or needling, was first applied to the distal portions of the limbs.

Classic of Bright Halls (*c.* 32 BC–106 AD)
The full development of the acupoints and acupuncture was achieved during the period immediately following the *Neijing*, and was marked by the compilation of the *Classic of Bright Halls*. The *Classic of Bright Halls*, which deals specifically with the acupoints, was compiled prior to 106 AD, between the latter part of the Western Han Dynasty (206 BC–24 AD) and the middle of the Eastern Han Dynasty (25–220 AD). Like the *Neijing* and many other classical texts, authorship of this classical medical document is attributed to Huang Di, the legendary Yellow Emperor. The book remained popular in the Sui (581–618 AD) and Tang (618–907 AD) Dynasties, when it was considered a primary medical textbook[11].

Although the original version of the *Classic of Bright Halls* was lost during the Northern Song Dynasty (960–1127 AD), around the time of the publication of *Illustrated Classic of Acupoints on the Bronze Model* (1027 AD)[12], its contents are well preserved in the *Systematic Classic of Acupuncture and Moxibustion* (*c.* 256–259 AD)[13]. Most of the material concerning acupuncture and moxibustion included in the *Classic of Bright Halls* was adapted from the *Neijing*, indicating that the *Neijing* preceded it and served as its primary source.

The *Neijing* and the later *Classic of Bright Halls* differ primarily in their selection of areas to be stimulated. The *Neijing* focuses on the general meridians, while the *Classic of Bright Halls* calls for stimulating specific acupoints, with a focus on those below the elbows and knees. For example, in cases of malaria with attacks every other day and no thirst, the *Neijing* calls for needling of the general Urinary Bladder Meridian of Foot Taiyang, while the *Classic of Bright Halls* selects UB60-Kunlun, a specific point on the Urinary Bladder Meridian. In cases of febrile disease in which pain first occurs in the forearm, the *Neijing* calls for needling the general Hand Yangming and Hand Taiyin Meridians, while the *Classic of Bright Halls* selects LU7-Lieque, a point on the Lung Meridian of Hand Taiyin[14].

In addition to reflecting the development of acupuncture from general meridians to specific acupoints, the *Classic of Bright Halls* reflects the theoretical and clinical development of the acupoints in the following areas.

First, there was a rapid increase in the discovery of new acupoints in the period immediately following the *Neijing*. The number of acupoints rose from 160 in the *Neijing* to 349 in the *Classic of Bright Halls*. This is an increase of 189 acupoints within less than 200 years. A mere twelve additional acupoints were added during the following 1600 years, to today's total of 361[15].

Second, acupoint theory made great progress. The *Neijing* mentions the five types of *shu* (transport) acupoints of eleven of the twelve Regular Meridians. The *Classic of Bright Halls* added not only the five *shu* (transport) acupoints of the twelfth Regular Meridian, the Heart Meridian, but also additional specific acupoints, including the *mu* (assembly), *xi* (cleft) and *jiaohui* (intersection) acupoints.

Third, indications of the acupoints were expanded. The *Neijing* calls primarily for moxibustion or needling of the general meridians, rather than specific acupoints. The *Classic of Bright Halls*, on the other hand, lists acupoints indicated for treatment of 270 diseases and disorders, including 185 internal conditions, twenty surgical conditions, twenty-three gynecological and pediatric conditions, and forty-two disorders of the five sensory organs[16].

A comparison of areas treated for four diseases in the four classical medical documents discussed above clearly shows the progression from stimulating general meridians to selecting specific acupoints. (See Table 3.2.)

A close investigation of the history of the meridians and acupoints indicates that the acupoints were not discovered prior to the meridians, as has generally been assumed. Rather, the identification of the meridians came first, and laid the necessary foundation for the identification of the acupoints.

The earliest medical documents, the *Medical Relics of Mawangdui* (*c.* prior to 168 BC), discuss treating the general meridians. The *Historical Records* (*c.* 104–91 BC) give cases of treating *suo* (areas) of the meridians, rather than their entire pathways; however, the emphasis is on the meridians, and no specific names or locations are given for the areas. For example, in cases of difficulty in urination, moxibustion is applied to bilateral *suo* (areas) of the Foot Jueyin Meridian. In cases of headache and fever, three bilateral *suo* (areas) of the Foot Yangming Meridian are needled. (See Table 3.2.)

The first mention of the acupoints occurs in the *Neijing* (*c.* 104–32 BC), which refers to them as *qixue* (caves of *qi*) or *qifu* (mansions of *qi*). They are defined as the areas where *qi* issues from the meridians. Chapter 59 of the *Suwen* section of the *Neijing*, entitled 'Discussion of *Qifu*', lists the approximate locations of the acupoints of a number of meridians, including the six Hand and Foot Yang Meridians and the Ren and Du Extraordinary Meridians. In each case, the acupoints are discussed in the

Table 3.2
Treatment of four diseases in four classical medical documents

Ailment	Medical Relics of Mawangdui (c. prior to 168 BC)	Historical Records (c. 104–91 BC)	Neijing (c. 104–32 BC)	Classic of Bright Halls (c. 32 BC–106 AD)
Toothache	Hand Yangming Meridian	Left Hand Yangming Meridian	Foot Yangming Meridian when there is preference for cold drinks, Hand Yangming Meridian when there is aversion to cold drinks; LI5-Pianli.	LI3-Sanjian, LI4-Hegu, LI5-Pianli, etc.
Retention of urine	Foot Jueyin Meridian	One *suo* (area) on each side of Foot Jueyin Meridian	Area posterior to nail of big toe	LR$_1$-Dadun
Deafness	Hand Shaoyang Meridian	No mention	Area posterior to nail of fourth finger	SJ1-Guanchong, SJ3-Zhongzhu, SJ5-Waiguan
Headache, fever and restlessness	Foot Yangming Meridian	Three *suo* (areas) on each side of Foot Yangming Meridian	Dorsal portion of Foot Yangming Meridian	ST44-Neiting

context of their meridians; for example, 'The Urinary Bladder Meridian of Foot Taiyang has seventy-eight acupoints from which its *qi* issues'[17].

From the earliest mention of acupoints in the ancient documents until their maturity at the time of the *Classic of Bright Halls* (c. 32 BC–106 AD), they have been considered to be integral parts of the meridians rather than discrete islets on the surface of the body[18]. They are generally located on specific areas of the meridians, including the bony holes or depressions in the bones; between the bones, muscles or tendons; around or on the joints of the limbs, such as wrist, elbow, shoulder, ankle and knee; near the arteries (referred to classically as the moving vessels); and above the hairline or on the extremities[19]. The *Classic of Bright Halls* uses the term *xian* (depression) to describe the anatomical characteristics of the acupoints. Just as water flows to depressions in the earth, so the *qi* and blood of the meridians converge in the areas of the acupoints.

Consequently, familiarity with the pathway of a meridian will enable the practitioner easily to locate its specific acupoints. The *Neijing* succinctly states[20]:

> There are a total of 365 acupoints. If one grasps the essentials of meridian theory, the numerous acupoints can be described with just one sentence. If one fails to grasp these essentials, the points will seem boundless.

When the body is out of balance, positive signs will usually appear along the pathways of the affected meridians. These signs, which may include soreness, tenderness, scleroma and changes in skin color, are generally located at or near acupoints. The *Neijing* stresses repeatedly that, before applying stimulation, the pathways of the affected meridians should always be examined and palpated in order to locate the exact acupoints. This practice is known as point diagnosis. It now becomes clear how the ancient Chinese discovered so many acupoints within such a short time. Once they had identified the pathways of the meridians and developed meridian theory, point diagnosis enabled them rapidly to determine the precise locations of the acupoints.

Finally, it is necessary to mention that the discovery of the acupoints was a direct result of the practice of acupuncture. While moxibustion can be applied to a large area of the body, or even along the entire course of a meridian, needles can only be inserted into the body through discrete points. The classical term for acupoint used in the *Neijing*, *qixue* (cave of *qi*), indicates that the acupoints are three-dimensional openings that allow the needles to be inserted into the body without injury to the tissues. Chapter 4 of the *Lingshu* states[21]:

> The acupuncturist should needle the *qixue* (caves of *qi*) and avoid the muscles. When the needle is inserted into the *qixue* (caves of *qi*), it is similar to moving through a lane or alley. There will be pain if the muscles are needled.

The close relation between the acupoints and acupuncture can be seen in this definition of the acupoints from the *Suwen*[22]:

> All three hundred and sixty-five *qixue* (caves of *qi*) are areas through which the needles enter the body.

The final piece in the puzzle of the historical development of acupuncture (literally 'acu-moxa therapy' in Chinese) thus falls into place. The Chinese ancestors first stimulated the body with moxibustion, and thereby identified the meridians. Only then did they develop the concept of acupuncture to stimulate specific sites along the meridians, gradually discovering the locations of the acupoints through meridian diagnosis. The correct chronological order of development of the four components of acupuncture is therefore moxibustion, meridians, acupuncture, and acupoints. (See Figure 1.2.)

Classification of the acupoints

There are numerous acupoints throughout the body. They are generally classified into three types: meridian acupoints, extraordinary acupoints, and *a-shi* ('oh yes') acupoints.

Meridian acupoints

Meridian acupoints, *jingxue* in Chinese, are those acupoints located along the pathways of the twelve Regular and two Extraordinary Meridians. Most of the 361 meridian acupoints in use today were discovered prior to the Western Jin Dynasty (265–316 AD), and might therefore properly be referred to as classical acupoints[23]. (See Table 3.3.) The acupoints of the twelve Regular Meridians are distributed symmetrically in pairs on the bilateral sides of the body, while those of the Ren and Du Extraordinary Meridians are located along single pathways, anterior and posterior to the vertical midline of the trunk respectively.

The names of the meridian acupoints contain significant meaning. The human body is a miniature of the universe, and the nomenclature of the acupoints reflects this holistic thinking. Distributed over the surface of the human body one will find mountains (GB40-Qiuxu, Hillock and UB60-Kunlun, Kunlun Mountain), rivers (KI3-Taixi, Great Stream), clouds (LU2-Yunmen, Cloud Gate), celestial bodies (DU23-Shangxing, Upper Star), plants (UB2-Cuanzhu, Bamboo Gathering), animals (ST35-Dubi, Calf's Nose), buildings (RN19-Zigong, Purple Palace) and utensils (ST12-Quepen, Broken Basin), among others.

Table 3.3
Number of meridian acupoints recorded at various historical stages

Reference	Single pathway acupoints	Bilateral acupoints	Total number of acupoints
Neijing (c. 104–32 BC)	25	135	160
Systematic Classic of Acupuncture and Moxibustion (c. 259 AD)	49	300	349
Illustrated Classic of Acupoints on the Bronze Model (1027 AD)	51	303	354
Compendium of Acupuncture (1601 AD)	51	308	359
Benefits of Acupuncture and Herbs (1815 AD)	52	309	361

Extraordinary acupoints

Extraordinary acupoints, *qixue* in Chinese, refer to acupoints that have specific names and definite locations, but are not subordinate to the meridians. 'Extraordinary' here has two meanings: first, most of these acupoints are not on the pathways of the twelve Regular and two Extraordinary Meridians; and secondly, many of them have specific effects. Although thousands of extraordinary acupoints have been established over the centuries, only about fifty are commonly used in the clinic today[24].

A-shi acupoints

A-shi means 'oh yes' in English. *A-shi* acupoints are determined by positive signs such as tenderness or scleroma, but are without fixed positions or names. They are also called unfixed points or tender points. *A-shi* acupoints are usually on or adjacent to diseased locations, and are used primarily for treatment of pain conditions. A number of *a-shi* acupoints that occur at fixed positions and are used frequently in the clinic have been named and classified as extraordinary acupoints.

Of these three types of acupoints, the meridian acupoints are the most important and most commonly used in clinical practice.

Effects of the acupoints

The effects of acupoints are quite different from those of medicinal herbs. The properties of herbs are generally fixed. For instance, a cooling herb can only be used to treat heat conditions. The effects of the acupoints, on the other hand, are directly related to the condition of the patient. Puncturing an acupoint will generally not produce any effect on a healthy person. In cases of disease or disorder, puncturing the same point in the same way may produce opposite effects depending on the condition being treated. For example, puncturing DU20-Baihui can excite the mind in cases of depression or drowsiness, or calm it in cases of mania or insomnia. Treating ST36-Zusanli can relax the stomach to treat gastric spasm, or strengthen it in cases of gastric flaccidity to stimulate peristalsis. Selecting PC6-Neiguan can either slow the heartbeat in cases of tachycardia, or quicken it in cases of bradycardia; DU14-Dazhui can lower the body temperature in cases of high fever, or warm the body when there is a low tolerance for cold.

This property of the acupoints is known as the bi-directional regulating effect. An acupoint may have either cooling or warming properties, depending on whether it is used for heat or cold conditions. In the same way, it may have either reducing or reinforcing properties, depending on whether it is used for excessive or deficient conditions. (See Chapter 4 for further discussion of the mechanics of the bi-directional effect.) The acupoints therefore cannot be categorized by property, since their properties vary according to condition. Rather, acupoints are usually subdivided according to the locations they affect – i.e. local, distal, sectional or specific.

Local effect

Local effect means that an acupoint is effective for problems that occur on or adjacent to its location. All acupoints, including the meridian, extraordinary and *a-shi* acupoints, have a local effect. For examples, acupoints around the eyes can all be used for eye problems; LI4-Hegu, on the back of the hand, is effective for conditions of the hands including pain, motor impairment and swelling; the extraordinary acupoint Ex-Yintang, located on the middle of the glabella, is effective for frontal headache, pain in the supraorbital region and nasal diseases. Acupoints on the head, face and neck have primarily local effect.

Sectional effect

Sectional effect means that an acupoint is effective for problems that occur in the horizontal cross-section in which it is located. Acupoints located on the trunk, especially those of the Ren and Du Meridians, as well as the front *mu* (assembly) and back *shu* (transport) acupoints of the internal *zangfu* organs, have a sectional effect. For instance, in addition to their local effect, the front *mu* (assembly) and back *shu* (transport) acupoints of each internal *zangfu* organ form a pair of points indicated for diseases and disorders of the organ. (See Table 3.4.) Sectional effect is usually included in the category of local effect in acupuncture texts, but I do think it is helpful in practice to distinguish them from each other.

Distal effect

Distal effect means that an acupoint is effective for problems that are far removed from its location. Many acupoints, especially those of the twelve Regular Meridians located below the elbow and knee, have a distal effect. In additional to local disorders, these acupoints can be used to treat problems on the head and trunk, or even general conditions. There are four 'command' (or primary) meridian acupoints with a distal effect: ST36-

Table 3.4
Indications of acupoints on the trunk

Location	Indications
Acupoints on the chest, upper back (T1–T7)	Disorders of the lungs and heart
Acupoints on the upper abdomen (above the umbilicus) and lower back (T8–L1)	Disorders of the liver, gallbladder, spleen and stomach
Acupoints on the lower abdomen (below the umbilicus) and lumbosacral region (L2–S4)	Disorders of the kidney, intestines, bladder, and genital organs

Zusanli is effective for problems of the abdomen, UB40-Weizhong for problems of the back, LU7-Lieque for disorders on the back of the neck, and LI4-Hegu for problems of the face and mouth, including toothache.

Specific effect

Specific effect means that an acupoint is effective for specific symptoms or diseases. Some meridian or extraordinary acupoints may have a specific effect. For example, DU14-Dazhui is effective for lowering high fever, RN4-Guanyuan is effective for general deficient conditions, Ex-Sifeng is used for infantile indigestion, and LI4-Hegu is used to treat pain conditions.

To summarize, all acupoints, including meridian, extraordinary and *a-shi* acupoints, have a local effect. Many acupoints on the trunk have a sectional effect, and many meridian and extraordinary acupoints, especially those below the elbows and knees, have a distal effect. Why is this so? To understand the different effects of the various acupoints, it is useful to subdivide them into two groups, i.e. Root acupoints and Tip acupoints. Root acupoints refer to acupoints on the limbs, which are the Roots of the meridians; Tip acupoints refer to acupoints on the trunk and head, which are the Tips of the meridians. The *Neijing* offers the following locations for some Root and Tip acupoints. (See Table 3.5.)

Table 3.5
Locations of Root and Tip acupoints of the Regular Meridians (based on Chapter 52 of the *Lingshu*)

Regular Meridians	Root acupoints	Tip acupoints
Foot Taiyang Meridian	5 *cun* above heel (approx. UB59-Fuyang)	Eye (approx. UB1-Jingming)
Foot Shaoyang Meridian	GB44-Zuqiaoyin	Anterior to ear (approx. GB2-Tinghui)
Foot Yangming Meridian	ST45-Lidui	ST9-Renying, cheek and nose
Foot Taiyin Meridian	4 *cun* superior and anterior to LR4-Zhongfeng (approx. SP6-Sanyinjiao)	UB20-Pishu, root of tongue
Foot Shaoyin Meridian	2 *cun* above inner joint of ankle (approx. KI8-Jiaoxin)	UB23-Shenshu, root of tongue
Foot Jueyin Meridian	5 *cun* above LR2-Xingjian (approx. LR4-Zhongfeng)	UB18-Ganshu
Hand Taiyang Meridian	Behind wrist (approx. SI5-Yanggu)	1 *cun* above eye (approx. UB2-Cuanzhu)
Hand Shaoyang Meridian	2 *cun* above web between fourth and fifth fingers (approx. SJ3-Zhongzhu)	Outer canthus (approx. SJ23-Sizhukong)
Hand Yangming Meridian	Elbow and back of upper arm (approx. LI11-Quchi, LI14-Binao)	Below mandible (approx. LI18-Futu)
Hand Taiyin Meridian	*Cukou* or wrist pulse (approx. LU9-Taiyuan)	Moving vessel (artery) anterior to axilla (approx. LU1-Zhongfu)
Hand Shaoyin Meridian	Head of ulna (approx. HT7-Shenmen)	UB15-Xinshu
Hand Jueyin Meridian	On medial side of forearm in depression between two tendons, 2 *cun* above crease of wrist (approx. PC6-Neiguan)	3 *cun* below axilla (approx. PC1-Tianchi)

Just as cultivating the roots of a tree causes its branches and leaves to flourish, so stimulating the Root acupoints, located on the limbs, or the Roots of the meridians, will not only activate the flow of *qi* and blood in the local areas, but also have a distal effect on the head and trunk. Conversely, stimulating the Tip acupoints, located on the trunk and head, or Tips of the meridians, will produce mainly local or sectional effects. Treating distal problems is one of the essential aspects of acupuncture, both verifying and embodying holistic thinking. Whenever we needle acupoints on the limbs to treat disorders on the head or trunk, we see holism in action.

Specific acupoints

Among the meridian acupoints are ten groups of specific acupoints, each group sharing common therapeutic properties. They are the five types of *shu* (transport) acupoints of the Regular Meridians, and the *yuan* (source), *luo* (connecting), back *shu* (transport), front *mu* (assembly), *xi* (cleft), lower *he* (convergence), *hui* (influential), *hui* (confluence) and *jiaohui* (intersection) acupoints. The specific acupoints are the most commonly used acupoints clinically. The majority of the specific acupoints are located on the limbs, the Roots of the meridians, primarily below the elbows and knees. The *jiaohui* (intersection) acupoints are the exception; they are located mainly on the head and trunk, the Tips of the meridians, since these are areas where the meridians usually intersect or overlap. Most of the specific acupoints were first recorded in the *Lingshu* section of the *Neijing*. (See Figure 3.1 and Table 3.6.)

Table 3.6
Distribution of specific acupoints (with exception of *jiaohui* (intersection) acupoints)

Location	Specific acupoints	Other acupoints	Total acupoints	Percentage of total
Head and neck	0	74	74	0
Trunk	29	110	139	20.9
Limbs (above elbows and knees)	1	33	34	2.9
Limbs (below elbows and knees)	99	15	114	86.8
Total	129	232	361	35.7

The five types of *shu* (transport) acupoints

The five types of *shu* (transport) acupoints are located on each of the twelve Regular Meridians, below the elbows or knees. From distal to proximal, they are the *jing* (well), *ying* (spring), *shu* (stream), *jing* (river) and *he* (sea) acupoints. (See Tables 3.7, 3.8.)

The five types of *shu* (transport) acupoints of the Regular Meridians are the most important specific acupoints clinically. As mentioned previously, the first acupoints to be discovered were those on the limbs. Of these original points, the five types of *shu* (transport) acupoints of the Regular Meridians were the first to be discussed in detail. The second chapter of the *Lingshu* (*c.* 104–32 BC) lists the names and locations of the five *shu* (transport) acupoints of eleven of the twelve Regular Meridians, omitting only those of the Heart Meridian. The *Classic of Bright Halls* (*c.* 32 BC–106 AD) adds the five *shu* (transport) acupoints of the Heart Meridian, bringing the total up to the current sixty[25].

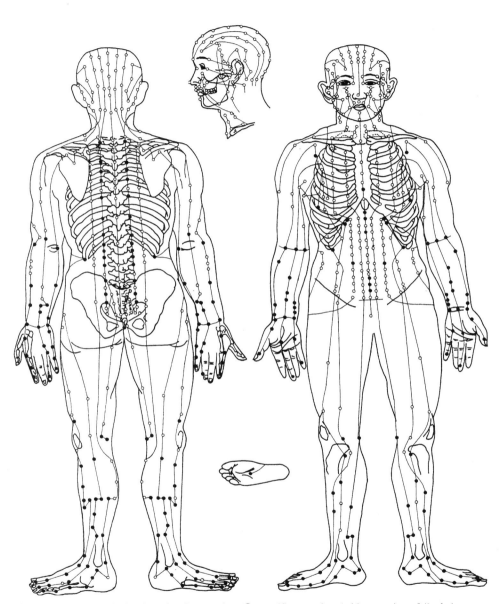

Figure 3.1   General distribution of main acupoints. ●: specific acupoints (with exception of *jiaohui* (intersection acupoints; ○: *jiaohui* (intersection) and other acupoints.

Table 3.7
Five types of *shu* (transport) acupoints of the Yin Regular Meridians and their corresponding elements

	Jing (well) wood	*Ying* (spring) fire	*Shu* (stream) earth	*Jing* (river) metal	*He* (sea) water
Lung Meridian	LU11-Shaoshang	LU10-Yuji	LU9-Taiyuan	LU8-Jingqu	LU5-Chize
Spleen Meridian	SP1-Yinbai	SP2-Dadu	SP3-Taibai	SP5-Shangqiu	SP9-Yinlingquan
Heart Meridian	HT9-Shaochong	HT8-Shaofu	HT7-Shenmen	HT4-Lingdao	HT3-Shaohai
Kidney Meridian	KI1-Yongquan	KI2-Rangu	KI3-Taixi	KI7-Fuliu	KI10-Yingu
Pericardium Meridian	PC9-Zhongchong	PC8-Laogong	PC7-Daling	PC5-Jianshi	PC3-Quze
Liver Meridian	LR1-Dadun	LR2-Xingjian	LR3-Taichong	LR4-Zhongfeng	LR8-Ququan

Table 3.8
Five types of *shu* (transport) acupoints of the Yang Regular Meridians and their corresponding elements

	Jing (well) metal	*Ying* (spring) water	*Shu* (stream) wood	*Jing* (river) fire	*He* (sea) earth
Large Intestine Meridian	LI1-Shangyang	LI2-Erjian	LI3-Sanjian	LI5-Yangxi	LI11-Quchi
Stomach Meridian	ST45-Lidui	ST44-Neiting	ST43-Xiangu	ST41-Jiexi	ST36-Zusanli
Small Intestine Meridian	SI1-Shaoze	SI2-Qiangu	SI3-Houxi	SI5-Yanggu	SI8-Xiaohai
Urinary Bladder Meridian	UB67-Zhiyin	UB66-Zutonggu	UB65-Shugu	UB60-Kunlun	UB40-Weizhong
San Jiao Meridian	SJ1-Guanchong	SJ2-Yemen	SJ3-Zhongzhu	SJ6-Zhigou	SJ10-Tianjing
Gallbladder Meridian	GB44-Zuqiaoyin	GB43-Xiaxi	GB41-Zulinqi	GB38-Yangfu	GB34-Yanglingquan

The *Nanjing* (*c.* prior to 25 AD) developed the theory of the five types of *shu* (transport) acupoints further.

The five types of *shu* (transport) acupoints reflect differences in the flow of *qi* and blood through the Regular Meridians. Although the flow of *qi* and blood through the interconnected system of meridians is circular, the quantity of the flow varies at different points. The amount of *qi* and blood is least at the ends of the limbs, which are the Roots or origin of the Regular Meridians. As the flow moves towards the head and trunk, which are the Tips or ends of the meridians, the amount of *qi* and blood increases. This progression resembles the flow of water along the course of a river. The *jing* (well) acupoint, at the tip of the finger or toe, is the point where the *qi* starts to bubble. At the *ying* (spring) acupoint, generally anterior to the metacarpophalangeal or metatarsophalangeal joint, the *qi* starts to gush. At the *shu* (stream) acupoint, generally posterior to the metacarpophalangeal or metatarsophalangeal joint or on the wrist or ankle, the *qi* moves briskly. At the *jing* (river) acupoint, usually on or above the wrist or ankle, the *qi* pours abundantly through the meridian. Finally, the *qi* reaches the *he* (sea) acupoint, on the elbow or knee, the point of confluence of the waters into the sea[26]. (See Figure 2.3.)

The five types of *shu* (transport) acupoints – *jing* (well), *ying* (spring), *shu* (stream), *jing* (river) and *he* (sea) – are widely used in the clinic. They are applied according to their properties and a number of different systems.

Acupoint properties
Each of the five types of *shu* (transport) acupoints has specific properties. The *jing* (well) acupoints function to clear heat and open the orifices. Due to their ease of access, the *jing* (well) acupoints of the six Hand Regular Meridians are usually used in combination to reduce fever and restore consciousness. The *ying* (spring) and *shu* (stream) acupoints of the Yang Regular Meridians can effectively quicken the flow of *qi* and blood, and are used to treat problems on the external pathways of these meridians. The *Lingshu* directs: 'Apply the *ying* (spring) or *shu* (stream) acupoints [of the Yang Regular Meridians] to treat problems on their external pathways'[27].

The *ying* (spring) acupoints of the Yin Regular Meridians also function to clear heat, and are used to cool fire within these meridians and their related *zang* organs. For instance, LR2-Xingjian, the *ying* (spring) acupoint of the Liver Meridian, is used to cool liver fire. The *shu* (stream) acupoints of the Yin Regular Meridians, also classified as *yuan* (source) acupoints, are effective for treating problems of these meridians' internally related *zang* organs. The *Suwen* states: 'In cases of problems of the *zang* organs, stimulate their *shu* (stream) acupoints'[28].

The *jing* (river) acupoints of both the Yin and Yang Regular Meridians function to dredge the meridians and collaterals. They are also used to treat problems on the external pathways of these meridians. The *he* (sea) acupoints of all Yin Regular Meridians and the Foot Yang Meridians are effective for treating diseases of these meridians' internally related *zangfu* organs. The *he* (sea) acupoints of the Hand Yang Regular Meridians, however, are used primarily for external problems. Problems of the internally related *fu* organs of these meridians are treated by stimulating their lower *he* (convergence) acupoints.

Five Elements Mother–Child relationships
According to Five Elements theory, 'Mother–Child' relationships exist among the five elements – wood, fire, earth, metal and water. The *Lingshu* records that each of the five types of *shu* (transport) acupoints corresponds to one of these elements, according to its meridian. The five types of *shu* (transport) acupoints of the Yin Regular Meridians – the *jing* (well), *ying* (spring), *shu* (stream), *jing* (river) and *he* (sea) points from distal to proximal – correspond to wood, fire, earth, metal and water respectively. Those of the Yang Regular Meridians – also *jing* (well), *ying* (spring), *shu* (stream), *jing* (river), and *he* (sea) points from distal to proximal – correspond to metal, water, wood, fire and earth respectively[29]. (See Tables 3.7, 3.8.)

The *Nanjing* (c. prior to 25 AD) directs practitioners to 'Supplement the Mother in cases of deficiency and reduce the Child in cases of excess', in accordance with Five Elements Theory[30]. For example, the lung corresponds to metal. Water is the Child of metal, so when the lung is excessive, LU5-Chize, which corresponds to water according to the Yin Meridian correspondences listed above, is stimulated using the reducing method. Earth is the Mother of metal, so when the lung is deficient, LU9-Taiyuan, which corresponds to earth according to the Yin Meridian correspondences listed above, is stimulated using the reinforcing method. (See Table 3.9.)

Table 3.9
Mother–Child *shu* (transport) acupoints of the *zangfu* organs and their corresponding elements

Zangfu organ and corresponding element	Mother *shu* (transport) acupoint and corresponding element	Child *shu* (transport) acupoint and corresponding element
Lung, metal	LU9-Taiyuan, *shu* (stream), earth	LU5-Chize, *he* (sea), water
Large Intestine, metal	LI11-Quchi, *he* (sea), earth	LI2-Erjian, *ying* (spring), water
Kidney, water	KI7-Fuliu, *jing* (river), metal	KI1-Yongquan, *jing* (well), wood
Urinary bladder, water	UB67-Zhiyin, *jing* (well), metal	UB65-Shugu, *shu* (stream), wood
Liver, wood	LR8-Ququan, *he* (sea), water	LR2-Xingjian, *ying* (spring), fire
Gallbladder, wood	GB43-Xiaxi, *ying* (spring), water	GB38-Yangfu, *jing* (river), fire
Heart, fire	HT9-Shaochong, *jing* (well), wood	HT7-Shenmen, *shu* (stream), earth
Small intestine, fire	SI3-Houxi, *shu* (stream), wood	SI8-Xiaohai, *he* (sea), earth
Pericardium, fire	PC9-Zhongchong, *jing* (well), wood	PC7-Daling, *shu* (stream), earth
San Jiao, fire	SJ3-Zhongzhu, *shu* (stream), wood	SJ10-Tianjing, *he* (sea), earth
Spleen, earth	SP2-Dadu, *ying* (spring), fire	SP5-Shangqiu, *jing* (river), metal
Stomach, earth	ST41-Jiexi, *jing* (river), fire	ST45-Lidui, *jing* (well), metal

The five types of *shu* (transport) points have very powerful effects, especially on their related internal *zangfu* organs. They are therefore sometimes called the *shu* (transport) points of the *zangfu* organs. The *Lingshu* states: 'Those points [i.e. the five types of *shu* (transport) acupoints] are points of the five *zang* and six *fu* organs'[31].

Midday–Midnight acupoint selection
The Chinese ancestors believed that, just like the waters of the sea, the flow of *qi* and blood within the meridians is influenced by the movement of the sun, moon and earth. The Midday–Midnight theory classifies and selects the five types of *shu* (transport) acupoints according to daily, monthly and yearly cycles. This theory originated at the time of the *Neijing* (c. 104–32 BC), but was not perfected until the Jin (1115–1234 AD) and Yuan (1271–1368 AD) Dynasties. Although this method may allow essentially accurate selection of acupoints, it is not popularly practiced today due to its complexity and inflexibility.

Yuan (source) acupoints

Each of the twelve Regular Meridians has one *yuan* (source) acupoint, located at or below the ankle or wrist. The *yuan* (source) acupoint of each Yin Regular Meridian overlaps with its *shu* (stream) acupoint (one of the five types of *shu* (transport) acupoints). The *yuan* (source) acupoints of the Yang Regular Meridians do not overlap with any other points. (See Table 3.10.)

The *yuan* (source) acupoints were first listed in the *Lingshu* (c. 104–32 BC)[32]. Their locations, at or below the ankle and wrist, correspond with the points of origin of the meridians listed in the two oldest texts on the meridians from Mawangdui. (See Appendices 2 and 3.) The *yuan* (source) acupoints are considered to be the points of origin of each of the twelve Regular Meridians.

The *yuan* (source) acupoints, especially those of the Yin Regular Meridians, are very important for both diagnosis and treatment of problems of their internally related *zang* organs. The *Lingshu* summarizes[33]:

Table 3.10
Yuan (source) and *luo* (connecting) acupoints of the twelve Regular Meridians

Regular Meridians	*Yuan* (source) acupoint	*Luo* (connecting) acupoint
Lung Meridian	LU9-Taiyuan	LU7-Lieque
Large Intestine Meridian	LI4-Hegu	LI6-Pianli
Stomach Meridian	ST42-Chongyang	ST40-Fenglong
Spleen Meridian	SP3-Taibai	SP4-Gongsun
Heart Meridian	HT7-Shenmen	HT5-Tongli
Small Intestine Meridian	SI4-Wangu	SI7-Zhizheng
Urinary Bladder Meridian	UB64-Jinggu	UB58-Feiyang
Kidney Meridian	KI3-Taixi	KI4-Dazhong
Pericardium Meridian	PC7-Daling	PC6-Neiguan
San Jiao Meridian	SJ4-Yangchi	SJ5-Waiguan
Gallbladder Meridian	GB40-Qiuxu	GB37-Guangming
Liver Meridian	LR3-Taichong	LR5-Ligou

In cases of problems of the five *zang* organs, select their respective *yuan* (source) acupoints . . . When there is illness in the five *zang* organs, there will be manifestations on their corresponding *yuan* (source) acupoints. Inspect the *yuan* (source) acupoints to determine the condition of the five *zang* organs.

Luo (connecting) acupoints

The *luo* (connecting) acupoints of each of the twelve Regular Meridians are located at the point where the meridian's collateral splits off from the main pathway, on the way to connect with its interior–exterior related meridian. Each Regular Meridian has a *luo* (connecting) acupoint. (See Table 3.10.) Additionally, the major collaterals of the Spleen, Ren and Du Meridians each have their own *luo* (connecting) acupoints: SP21-Dabao, RN15-Jiuwei, and DU1-Changqiang respectively. There is therefore a total of fifteen *luo* (connecting) acupoints.

The *luo* (connecting) acupoints were first listed in the *Lingshu* (*c.* 104–32 BC)[34]. The collaterals, especially those of the twelve Regular Meridians, connect each pair of interior–exterior related meridians. The *luo* (connecting) acupoints can therefore be used to treat problems of interior–exterior related meridians. For example, the Stomach and Spleen Meridians are interior–exterior related. The *luo* (connecting) acupoint of the Stomach Meridian, ST40-Fenglong, can therefore strengthen both the spleen and stomach, and is effective for phlegm conditions due to dysfunction of the spleen. Conversely, the *luo* (connecting) acupoint of the Spleen Meridian SP4-Gongsun quickens the flow of *qi* and blood, and is used to relieve stomachache.

The *luo* (connecting) and *yuan* (source) acupoints of the Regular Meridians are often used in combination. Because each pair of interior–exterior meridians are closely related, pathological conditions of one tend to affect the other. If both of a pair of interior–exterior meridians are diseased, the *yuan* (source) acupoint of the initially affected meridian and the *luo* (connecting) acupoint of the secondarily affected meridian are generally treated together. For instance, if a patient initially suffers from a lung problem and later becomes constipated, LU9-Taiyuan, the *yuan* (source) acupoint of the Lung Meridian, and LI6-Pianli, the *luo* (connecting) acupoint of the Large Intestine Meridian, are used in combination.

Table 3.11
Back *shu* (transport) and front *mu* (assembly) acupoints of the *zangfu* organs

Zangfu organ	Back *shu* (transport) acupoint	Front *mu* (assembly) acupoint
Lung	UB13-Feishu	LU1-Zhongfu
Large intestine	UB25-Dachangshu	ST25-Tianshu
Stomach	UB21-Weishu	RN12-Zhongwan
Spleen	UB20-Pishu	LR13-Zhangmen
Heart	UB15-Xinshu	RN14-Juque
Small intestine	UB27-Xiaochangshu	RN4-Guanyuan
Urinary bladder	UB28-Pangguangshu	RN3-Zhongji
Kidney	UB23-Shenshu	GB25-Jingmen
Pericardium	UB14-Jueyinshu	RN17-Danzhong
San Jiao	UB22-Sanjiaoshu	RN5-Shimen
Gallbladder	UB19-Danshu	GB24-Riyue
Liver	UB18-Ganshu	LR14-Qimen

Back *shu* (transport) acupoints

The back *shu* (transport) acupoints are located on the back of the trunk at the points where the *qi* and blood of the internal *zangfu* organs converge and disperse. There is a total of twelve back *shu* (transport) acupoints, one for each of the *zangfu* organs. They are all located on the first line of the Urinary Bladder Meridian on the back. (See Table 3.11.)

The back *shu* (transport) acupoints were first listed in the *Lingshu* (*c.* 104–32 BC)[35]. They are important for treating disorders of their corresponding *zangfu* organs, as well as problems of their *zangfu* organs' related tissues. For example, the liver opens into the eyes, so UB18-Ganshu, the back *shu* (transport) acupoint of the liver, can be used to treat various eye troubles. Clinically, the back *shu* (transport) acupoints are usually used in combination with their front *mu* (assembly) acupoints.

The back *shu* (transport) acupoints are important for diagnosing, as well as treating, problems of the *zangfu* organs and their related tissues. When the *zangfu* organs or their related tissues are diseased there will usually be positive reactions, such as tenderness or scleroma, on their corresponding back *shu* (transport) acupoints. The *Lingshu* states[36]:

> Press the back *shu* (transport) acupoint to confirm diagnosis. There will be tenderness when the back *shu* (transport) acupoint is pressed; the pain inside may be relieved immediately if the exact spot is found.

Front *mu* (assembly) acupoints

The front *mu* (assembly) acupoints are located on the front of the trunk at the points where the *qi* and blood of the internal *zangfu* organs converge and disperse. There is a total of twelve front *mu* (assembly) acupoints, one for each of the *zangfu* organs. (See Table 3.11.)

The front *mu* (assembly) acupoints were first listed in the *Classic of Bright Halls* (*c.* 32 BC–106 AD). They are important for both the diagnosis and treatment of problems of their related *zangfu* organs, and are usually used in combination with their corresponding back *shu* (transport) acupoints.

Table 3.12
Sixteen *xi* (cleft) acupoints of interior–exterior related meridians

Yin Meridians (interior)	*Xi* (cleft) acupoint	*Xi* (cleft) acupoint	Yang Meridians (exterior)
Lung Meridian	LU6-Kongzui	LI7-Wenliu	Large Intestine Meridian
Spleen Meridian	SP8-Diji	ST34-Liangqiu	Stomach Meridian
Heart Meridian	HT6-Yinxi	SI6-Yanglao	Small Intestine Meridian
Kidney Meridian	KI5-Shuiquan	UB63-Jinmen	Urinary Bladder Meridian
Pericardium Meridian	PC4-Ximen	SJ7-Huizong	San Jiao Meridian
Liver Meridian	LR6-Zhongdu	GB36-Waiqiu	Gallbladder Meridian
Yinwei Meridian	KI9-Zhubin	GB35-Yangjiao	Yangwei Meridian
Yinqiao Meridian	KI8-Jiaoxin	UB59-Fuyang	Yangqiao Meridian

Xi (cleft) acupoints

The *xi* (cleft) acupoints are a group of deep acupoints located on the limbs, primarily below the knees and elbows, where the flow of *qi* and blood converges. There is a total of sixteen *xi* (cleft) acupoints, one on each Regular Meridian and one each on the Yinqiao, Yangqiao, Yinwei and Yangwei Extraordinary Meridians. (See Table 3.12.)

The *xi* (cleft) acupoints were first listed in the *Classic of Bright Halls* (*c.* 32 BC–106 AD). Because the *xi* (cleft) acupoints are points of deep convergence of the *qi* and blood of the meridians, they are effective for quickening the flow of *qi* and blood and treating acute problems and severe pain along their related meridians. For example, ST34-Liangqiu, the *xi* (cleft) acupoint of the Stomach Meridian, is used for acute stomachache; PC4-Ximen, the *xi* (cleft) acupoint of the Pericardium Meridian, is effective for heart pain.

Lower *he* (convergence) acupoints

The six lower *he* (convergence) acupoints are located on the lower leg around the knee joint. Three are located on the Foot Yangming Meridian, two on the Foot Taiyang Meridian and one on the Foot Shaoyang Meridian. Each point corresponds to one of the six *fu* organs. The lower *he* (convergence) acupoints of the stomach, gallbladder and urinary bladder, ST36-Zusanli, GB34-Yanglingquan, and UB40-Weizhong respectively, are the same as the *he* (sea) acupoints of these *fu* organs' related meridians. The lower *he* (convergence) acupoints of the large intestine, small intestine and San Jiao are ST37-Shangjuxu, ST39-Xiajuxu, and UB39-Weiyang respectively.

The lower *he* (convergence) acupoints, especially those of the stomach, gallbladder and large intestine, are valuable in diagnosing and treating problems of the *fu* organs. There will usually be tenderness on these points when the related *fu* organs are affected. These points were first listed in the *Lingshu* (*c.* 104–32 BC), which states: 'Apply lower *he* 'convergence' acupoints to treat disorders of the six *fu* organs'[37]. They are usually used in combination with their corresponding front *mu* (assembly) acupoints. For example, ST37-Shangjuxu and ST25-Tianshu, the lower *he* (convergence) and front *mu* (assembly) acupoints of the large intestine, are an important pair of acupoints for almost all problems of the large intestine.

Table 3.13
Eight *hui* (influential) acupoints and their related tissues

Hui (influential) acupoints	Tissues
LR13-Zhangmen	*Zang* organs
RN12-Zhongwan	*Fu* organs
RN17-Danzhong	*Qi*
UB17-Geshu	Blood
GB34-Yanglingquan	Tendons
LU9-Taiyuan	Vessels
GB39-Xuanzhong	Marrow
UB11-Dazhu	Bones

Hui (influential) acupoints

There are eight *hui* (influential) acupoints, each of which has a specific influence upon one of the eight kinds of tissues – i.e. *zang* organs, *fu* organs, *qi*, blood, tendons, vessels, bones and marrow. (See Table 3.13.)

The *hui* (influential) acupoints were first listed in the *Nanjing* (*c.* prior to 25 AD)[38]. They are very important for both diagnosis and treatment of problems of their related tissues. For example, RN17-Danzhong, the *hui* (influential) acupoint of *qi*, is effective for quickening and supplementing the flow of *qi*, so it is a main acupoint for treating *qi* stagnation or deficiency.

Hui (confluence) acupoints of the eight Extraordinary Meridians

The eight *hui* (confluence) acupoints were discovered rather late in the development of acupuncture, during the Jin (1115–1234 AD) and Yuan (1271–1368 AD) Dynasties.

There are eight *hui* (confluence) acupoints, each of which is effective for treating disorders of one of the eight Extraordinary Meridians. They are located on the arms and legs, on eight of the twelve Regular Meridians – the Spleen, Pericardium, Small Intestine, Urinary Bladder, Gallbladder, San Jiao, Lung and Kidney Meridians.

In some cases, there is a direct connection between the Regular Meridian on which the *hui* (confluence) acupoint is located and the Extraordinary Meridian for which it is effective. For instance, UB62-Shenmai and KI6-Zhaohai, the *hui* (confluence) points of the Yangqiao and Yinqiao Meridians respectively, are located on the Urinary Bladder and Kidney Regular Meridians at the points where the Yangqiao and Yinqiao Extraordinary Meridians originate. LU7-Lieque, the *hui* (confluence) acupoint of the Ren Extraordinary Meridian, is located on the Lung Meridian; the Lung Regular Meridian and the Ren Extraordinary Meridian both connect with the throat.

However, in most cases there is no such direct connection. Rather, the effectiveness of most *hui* (confluence) acupoints has been revealed through clinical experience. For example, SI3-Houxi, the *hui* (confluence) acupoint of the Du Meridian, has been found to be effective for treating problems of the Du Meridian, such as backache and stiff neck, although there is no apparent connection between the Small Intestine Regular Meridian and the Du Extraordinary Meridian.

In addition to being applied singly, the *hui* (confluence) acupoints of the upper and lower limbs are usually applied in pairs. The four pairs of acupoints are used for the following four groups of conditions. (See Table 3.14.)

Table 3.14
Four pairs of *hui* (confluence) acupoints, their related Extraordinary Meridians and indications

Hui (confluence) acupoints and related Extraordinary Meridians	*Indications*
SP4-Gongsun (Chong Meridian), PC6-Neiguan (Yinwei Meridian)	Problems of the stomach, heart, and chest
SI3-Houxi (Du Meridian), UB62-Shenmai (Yangqiao Meridian)	Problems of the inner canthus, neck, ear and shoulder
GB41-Zulinqi (Dai Meridian), SJ5-Waiguan (Yangwei Meridian)	Problems of the outer canthus, posterior to the auricle, cheek, neck, and shoulder
LU7-Lieque (Ren Meridian), KI6-Zhaohai (Yinqiao Meridian)	Problems of the lungs, throat, trachea, chest and diaphragm

Jiaohui (intersection) acupoints

As the name implies, the *jiaohui* (intersection) acupoints refer to acupoints located at the intersection of two or more meridians. They are located mainly on the trunk and head, as the meridians usually overlap or intersect at these areas.

The *jiaohui* (intersection) acupoints were first mentioned in the *Lingshu* (*c.* 104–32 BC) and discussed more fully in the *Classic of Bright Halls* (*c.* 32 BC–106 AD). The *jiaohui* (intersection) acupoints can be used to treat problems of the various meridians that pass through them. There are many intersection acupoints, but only a limited number are useful in the clinic. (See Table 3.15.)

Table 3.15
Important *jiaohui* (intersection) acupoints

Acupoints	*Intersecting Meridians*
RN3-Zhongji	Ren Meridian, three Foot Yin Meridians
RN4-Guanyuan	Ren Meridian, three Foot Yin Meridians
RN12-Zhongwan	Ren Meridian, Hand and Foot Yangming Meridians, Hand Shaoyang Meridian
RN24-Chengjiang	Ren and Du Meridians, Hand and Foot Yangming Meridians
DU14-Dazhui	Du Meridian, all Hand and Foot Yang Meridians
DU20-Baihui	Du Meridian, Foot Jueyin Meridian, all Hand and Foot Yang Meridians
DU26-Shuigou	Du Meridian, Hand and Foot Yangming Meridians
LU1-Zhongfu	Hand and Foot Taiyin Meridians
SP6-Sanyinjiao	Three Foot Yin Meridians
UB62-Shenmai	Urinary Bladder and Yangqiao Meridians
KI6-Zhaohai	Kidney and Yinqiao Meridians
SJ20-Jiaosun	Hand and Foot Shaoyang Meridians
GB20-Fengchi	Gallbladder and Yangwei Meridians
GB26-Daimai	Gallbladder and Dai Meridians
GB30-Huantiao	Foot Shaoyang, Foot Taiyang Meridians
LR13-Zhangmen	Foot Jueyin, Foot Shaoyang Meridians
LR14-Qimen	Three Foot Yin Meridians

Acupoint diagnosis

The meridians unite the internal and the external and the upper and the lower parts of the body, linking it into an organic whole. When meridians or their related *zangfu* organs or tissues are diseased there will usually be manifestations along their external pathways, especially in the acupoint regions. Therefore, when diagnosing illness it is helpful to observe what is happening in the vicinity of the acupoints.

Diagnosis of illness

Like meridian diagnosis, acupoint diagnosis uses four techniques (inspection, palpation, measurement of skin electrical resistance and sensitivity to burning) to look for positive signs, including discoloration, deformities, desquamation, swollen blood vessels, tenderness, nodes and lowered electrical resistance. The only difference is that acupoint diagnosis concentrates on the acupoint regions, while meridian diagnosis focuses on the pathways of the meridians. Although positive signs may occur in areas that have no acupoints, or manifest on sections or even along the entire course of a meridian, the majority tend to occur in acupoint regions. Positive signs most commonly occur in the vicinity of the various types of specific acupoints, including the five types of *shu* (transport) acupoints, and the *xi* (cleft), *yuan* (source), *hui* (influential), back *shu* (transport) and front *mu* (assembly) acupoints. Therefore, particular attention should be paid to the specific acupoints when carrying out both meridian and acupoint diagnosis. (For discussion of meridian diagnosis, see Chapter 2.)

Verification of pattern identification

Acupoint diagnosis is usually not undertaken solely for the purpose of establishing a diagnosis. In fact, the practitioner may already have arrived at a complete understanding of the patient's condition and identified its pattern prior to undertaking acupoint diagnosis. In cases such as this, acupoint diagnosis can verify whether the pattern has been correctly identified. For example, take a case of vomiting. If the condition has been identified as an attack on the stomach by hyperactive liver *qi*, the acupoints of the Liver Meridian and the back *shu* (transport) acupoint of the liver (UB18-Ganshu) should be inspected. If positive signs are found on these acupoints, the identification is correct. However, if there is no reaction, the pattern identification may not be correct and should be reconsidered. This measure is especially useful in cases that have been treated repeatedly without improvement.

Determination of acupoint position

The areas where positive signs occur are the precise areas that should be stimulated to achieve optimum therapeutic results. They are similar to triggers – even mild or moderate stimulation will evince a strong needling sensation, with subsequent good therapeutic results. Due to individual differences, the location of positive signs may vary slightly from standard acupoint positions. For example, in cases of gallstone, tenderness is usually found 0.8–1.0 *cun* below GB34-Yanglingquan. This tender point is now considered to be an extraordinary acupoint, and is called EX-Dannangxue.

   Detection of positive signs through acupoint diagnosis is essential to determine the precise position of acupoints selected for treatment. The *Neijing* repeatedly recommends first pressing the acupoint, and only puncturing it if the patient feels sensations of tenderness or relief. This is particularly true when puncturing the specific acupoints, including back *shu* (transport), front *mu* (assembly), *xi* (cleft), and the five types of *shu* (transport) acupoints.

Evaluation of treatment

Finally, point diagnosis is valuable for evaluating therapeutic results. As the condition improves, positive signs will decrease and finally disappear. Acupoint diagnosis therefore enables the practitioner to identify whether or not there has been improvement, and how much.

Notes and References

1. *Lingshu*, 2:4–8; *Suwen*, 58–60:291–326.
2. *Suwen*, 58:291
3. *Lingshu*, 22:58.
4. *Ibid.*, 26:63.
5. *Ibid.*, 26:64.
6. *Ibid.*, 23:61
7. *Ibid.*, 24:62
8. *Ibid.*, 28:68
9. *Suwen*, 36:207
10. *Lingshu*, 2:4–8; *Suwen*, 58–59:291–317.
11. 'Bright Hall', or *mingtang* (明堂), originally referred to a building where the emperors, starting with Emperor Wu Di (*c.* 140 BC) of the Western Han Dynasty (206 BC–24 AD) promulgated their decrees. There were a total of twelve Bright Halls, one corresponding to each month of the year. The Emperor lived in each hall in turn for one month, rotating through all twelve halls over the course of a year. In the same way, each of the twelve Regular Meridians was considered to correspond to a month, and the flow of *qi* and blood through the interconnected system of twelve Regular Meridians to the progress of the 12 months of the year. Furthermore, acupoints were selected according to the waxing and waning of the moon. Thanks to these correspondences the term 'Bright Halls' gradually became a synonym for acupoints, and acupoint charts were called Maps of Bright Halls (*mingtang tu* 明堂图). Of the many books on acupoints named in this way, the *Classic of Bright Halls* is the oldest. See *Compilation and Annotation of the Yellow Emperor's Classic of Bright Halls* (*Huang Di Mingtangjing Jijiao* 黄帝明堂经辑校) (*c.* 32 BC–106 AD.) (ed. Huang Longxiang). Beijing: Chinese Medicine and Science Press, 1987, pp. 239–240.
12. *The Illustrated Classic of Acupoints on the Bronze Model* (*Tongren Shuxue Zhenjiu Tu Jing* 铜人腧穴针灸图经) was written by Wang Weiyi (987–1607 AD) in 1027 AD and engraved on stone. Bronze models that illustrated the acupoints discussed in the book were used as aids for teaching acupuncture. See Guo Shiyu, *History of Chinese Acupuncture and Moxibustion* (*Zhongguo Zhenjiu Shi* 中国针灸史). Tianjin: Tianjin Science and Technology Press, 1989, pp. 152–157.
13. *The Systematic Classic of Acupuncture and Moxibustion*, also translated as *The ABC of Acupuncture and Moxibustion* (*c.* 256–259 AD) (*Zhenjiu Jiayi Jing* 针灸甲乙经), compiled by Huangfu Mi (215–282 AD) during the Wei Dynasty (220–265 AD), is the earliest complete work on acupuncture and moxibustion extant in China. It contains material on acupuncture and moxibustion adapted from the *Neijing* and *Classic of Bright Halls*, and reflects the state of acupuncture and moxibustion at the time of the Wei Dynasty.
14. For details, see *Compilation and Annotation of Huang Di's Classic of Bright Halls*, pp. 272–286.
15. This total does not include the extraordinary or *a-shi* acupoints. (See Table 3.3.)

16. *Compilation and Annotation of Huang Di's Classic of Bright Halls*, p. 265.
17. *Suwen*, 59:303.
18. The theory of acupoints further developed with the much later discovery of the extraordinary and *a-shi* acupoints. The extraordinary acupoints are so called because they are generally not located on the pathways of meridians. (See discussion of extraordinary and *a-shi* acupoints in this chapter.)
19. The *Neijing* also refers to acupoints as *gukong* or empty spaces of the bones. Chapter 60 of the *Suwen*, 'Discussion of Empty Spaces of the Bones', lists a number of acupoints located in bony holes or between the bones, including UB31–34 Baliao, LI15-Jianyu, UB60-Kunlun, DU16-Fengfu (*Suwen*, 60:318–326.)
20. *Lingshu*, 1:3.
21. *Ibid.*, 4:15.
22. *Suwen*, 58:301.
23. I feel that it would be appropriate to add four additional extraordinary acupoints to this total, in order to increase the number of classical acupoints to 365 to correspond to the 365 days of the year, as stated in the *Neijing*. My suggested additions are: Ex-Yintang, on the course of the Du Meridian; Ex-Taiyang, on the course of the Gallbladder Meridian; Ex-Yishu, on the course of the Urinary Bladder Meridian; and Ex-Jianqian, on the course of the Lung Meridian.
24. For locations and indications of commonly used extraordinary acupoints, see Bai Xinghua *et al.*, *Acupuncture in Clinical Practice*. Oxford: Butterworth-Heinemann, 1996.
25. See Yang Shangshan (610–682 AD), *The Yellow Emperor's Inner Classic of Medicine: The Great Simplicity* (*Huang Di Neijing Taisu* 黄帝内经太素) (*c.* 650 AD). Beijing: People's Health Press, 1965, p.172. This is the oldest extant version of the *Neijing*, annotated *c.* 650 AD by Yang Shangshan (610–682 AD). It utilizes extensive material from the *Classic of Bright Halls* to annotate both the *Lingshu* and *Suwen*. Twenty-three of the thirty original chapters are still extant.
26. In addition to the five types of *shu* (transport) acupoints, a second system is also used to describe the concentric flow of *qi* and blood through the meridians. In this system, *gen* (root) refers to the *jing* (well) acupoints, *liu* (flowing) to the *yuan* (source) acupoints, *zhu* (pouring) to the *jing* (river) acupoints, and *ru* (entering) to two areas, one on the neck and the other at the *luo* (connecting) acupoints of each Regular Meridian. (See Table 3.16.)

Table 3.16
Gen (root), liu (flowing), zhu (pouring), and ru (entering) points of the six Yang Meridians (based on Chapter 5 of the Lingshu)

Yang Meridians	*Gen* (root)	*Liu* (flowing)	*Zhu* (pouring)	*Ru* (entering)	
				Lower	Upper
Foot Taiyang Meridian	UB67-Zhiyin	UB64-Jinggu	UB60-Kunlun	UB58-Feiyang	UB10-Tianzhu
Foot Shaoyang Meridian	GB44-Zuqiaoyin	GB40-Qiuxu	GB38-Yangfu	GB37-Guangming	SI17-Tianrong
Foot Yangming Meridian	ST45-Lidui	ST42-Chongyang	ST36-Zusanli	ST40-Fenglong	ST9-Renying
Hand Taiyang Meridian	SI1-Shaoze	SI5-Yanggu	SI10-Xiaohai	SI7-Zhizheng	SI16-Tianchuang
Hand Shaoyang Meridian	SJ1-Guanchong	SJ4-Yangchi	SJ6-Zhigou	SJ5-Waiguan	SJ16-Tianyou
Hand Yangming Meridian	LI1-Shangyang	LI4-Hegu	LI5-Yangxi	LI6-Pianli	LI18-Futu

27. *Lingshu*, 4:14.
28. *Suwen*, 38:217.
29. *Lingshu*, 2:4.
30. *Nanjing*, 69:35.
31. *Lingshu*, 2:7.
32. *Ibid.*, 1:3; 2:5.
33. *Ibid.*, 1:3.
34. *Ibid.*, 10:37.
35. *Ibid.*, 51:100.
36. *Ibid.*, 51:100.
37. *Ibid.*, 4:14.
38. *Nanjing*, 45:25.

Chapter 4
Acupuncture in practice – a holistic sculpture

'Acupuncture does not take effect unless there is *qizhi* or arrival of *qi*.'
Lingshu

The holistic interaction of practitioner, patient and needle

Clinically, the primary difference between drug therapy and acupuncture lies in the method of treatment. In drug therapy, the doctor prescribes medication and the patient takes it. The doctor may have no further contact with the patient after prescribing. The patient, in turn, simply takes the medication and hopes for the best. The doctor, the drug, the patient and the patient's body are four distinct entities, interacting across a gulf of objectification.

This limited interaction is not sufficient in acupuncture, in which practitioners not only prescribe acupoints but also have hands-on contact and interaction with their patients as they needle them repeatedly throughout the course of treatment. This is one reason why many practitioners of acupuncture, when asked to discuss their treatments, will expound at length upon their needling skills, and the size, shape and materials of their needles. However, acupuncturists, for all their pride in technique, can't pretend that they are single-handedly healing their patients. Consider for example infectious diseases. Acupuncture has been applied to treat infectious diseases since its invention. At the time of the *Neijing*, acupuncture was used for influenza, malaria, *bi* syndrome (including rheumatoid arthritis), and suppurative skin diseases such as furuncle and carbuncle. Yet bare metal needles obviously can't kill microbes directly.

How, then, is it possible for acupuncture to have an antimicrobial effect? It must be the patient's own body that kills the microbes. The most that acupuncture can claim for itself is that it promotes the body's self-healing powers. Modern understanding of the immunological functions within the human body supports this theory. Experiments show that acupuncture on humans with dysentery can stimulate and strengthen the body's humoral and cellular immunity, producing a marked increase in immunoglobulin, total complements, specific antibodies, fecal SIgA, the bactericidal properties of plasma, and phagocytic function[1].

Further evidence that acupuncture merely stimulates the body's innate powers of self-healing is provided by the bi-directional beneficial effects of some acupoints. As discussed in Chapter 3, some acupoints can cool and warm the same part of the body, or excite and inhibit the same function, depending upon the condition being treated. If acupuncture were merely a matter of technique, the same stimulus would always produce a consistent response. The human body, however, is far more subtle than that. The bi-directional effect is a reflection of the body's ability to achieve and maintain balance through a highly automatic control system dominated by Yin and Yang (☯), the receptive and active energies that compose the universe. These two opposites are fundamental to every facet of traditional Chinese medicine. The constantly changing balance that they embody may be seen in terms of modern medicine in the interaction between excitement and inhibition in the central nervous system, the relationship of the sympathetic and parasympathetic nervous systems, the balance of tropic and inhibitory hormones, and so on.

In a state of health, Yin and Yang condition each other. They regulate themselves automatically to adapt to changes in the internal and external environments so that all physiological functions stay in dynamic balance and the body functions at its peak. This is called homeostasis in modern medicine. However, if Yin and Yang fail to adapt to changes and maintain balance, there will be illness. The effectiveness of acupuncture lies in its ability to promote the body's automatic ability to reharmonize its activities, so that deficiency is supplemented, excess is reduced, cold is warmed, heat is cooled, excitation is inhibited, depression is excited, etc.

The natural power of the body to heal itself, referred to in this book as the self-healing force, is called *zheng qi* (正气) or right *qi* in traditional Chinese medicine. In terms of modern medicine, this self-healing force may include the functions of the nerves, the endocrine glands and the immune system, as well as functions that are still unknown. Illness is a result of the struggle between the body's self-healing force, or right *qi*, and pathogens, referred to as *xie qi* (邪气) or evil *qi* in TCM. The outcome of the fight depends upon the relative strength of the self-healing force and the pathogens. The condition will take a favorable turn if the self-healing force is strong and overcomes the pathogens; conversely, if the self-healing force is weak or the pathogens are too strong, the self-healing force will be defeated and there will be a change for the worse.

The strength of the self-healing force is related to many factors, including heredity, age, diet, exercise, occupation, lifestyle and environment. A person will be healthy if the self-healing force is powerful, and even if illness occurs the prognosis will be good. The *Neijing* states: 'If there is sufficiency of right *qi* inside, the evil *qi* can not invade'[2]. This is the reason that, although we are all surrounded by many pathogens, only a few of us become ill[3]. Only those whose self-healing force is weak will be susceptible to attack by pathogens. As the *Neijing* says: 'For evil *qi* to encroach, the right *qi* must be insufficient'[4].

Whenever the body is attacked, the self-healing force will automatically rise to meet the occasion and defeat the pathogens. In many cases, it will eventually be victorious with no outside assistance. For instance, most people will recover from a case of the common cold within a week. However, additional treatment can shorten the course of a cold considerably. With proper treatment, the manifestations may disappear within one day, several hours, or even immediately.

In many cases, however, especially chronic conditions, it will take a very long time to achieve a natural cure. In some cases there may never be a cure if no treatment is given. This indicates that it is not sufficient to depend upon the body's self-healing force alone to restore the body's balance. Application of an external force is necessary to assist the self-healing force. Acupuncture is just such a powerful force.

Acupuncture functions to cure disease and restore imbalance by arousing and strengthening the body's self-healing force. It stimulates a wide range of self-healing mechanisms inherent in the body, causing changes in almost all the physiological systems, including respiratory, digestive, cardiovascular, urogenital, musculoskeletal, nervous, endocrinal and immunological. When treating disease with acupuncture, the patient's own self-healing force is primary. The stimulation the practiner provides by needling is secondary, functioning to effectively catalyze and promote the natural rebalancing process.

The primary role of the self-healing force in acupuncture is indicated by the necessity of the patient's active participation in the treatment process. Acupuncture cannot be effectively administered without verbal feedback from the patient during treatment. It is essential that the practitioner ask the patient whether or not the needling sensation is being achieved during the course of needling.

Needling sensation, referred to as *qizhi* (arrival of *qi*) or *deqi* (obtaining *qi*) in the *Neijing*, is the subjective sensation experienced by the patient in response to effective needling stimulation. It may include feelings of localized soreness, heaviness, numbness or distension, or transmission of sensations upward or downward along the pathways of the meridians. Good therapeutic results will be obtained only if the needling sensation is achieved. The stronger the needling sensation the better the results will be, with the best results occurring if the needling sensation is experienced in the diseased area. The *Lingshu* states[5]:

> The essential point of acupuncture is to induce arrival of *qi*. Treatment will be effective only if there is arrival of *qi*. The effect obtained following arrival of *qi* is as visible as when a strong wind scatters the last clouds and the overcast sky suddenly becomes clear.

The *Ode of Golden Needles* further clarifies[6]:

> Immediate arrival of *qi* suggests that treatment will have a quick effect; delayed arrival of *qi* indicates that treatment will have a slow effect.

Achievement of the needling sensation is the sole indication of whether or not acupuncture treatment will be effective. Some practitioners think that the strength of the needling sensation is proportional to the force of needling, and that the more forceful the needling, the stronger the needling sensation will be. In fact, mild stimulation may lead to very strong needling sensation, while conversely there may be no sensation at all no matter how forceful the needling stimulation. This indicates that the patient's own self-healing force is of primary importance in obtaining the needling sensation, and that the needling stimulation is merely a catalyst.

Acupuncture is only one method for stimulating the body's self-healing force. Because it may seem rather frightening, over the ages practitioners have developed a number of less traumatic methods of stimulation for the benefit of their patients. These include acupressure, dry cupping and medicinal compresses, as well as modern needleless acupuncture using electrical, laser or magnetic stimulation. New methods of stimulating the acupoints continue to be developed. Although each of these methods has its own advantages and indications, none has been able to replace needling therapy. The reason might be that only traumatic stimulation can activate the body's maximum potential healing force.

A study on plants provides support for this hypothesis. Scientists at the University of California demonstrated that a certain amount of damage to a plant's leaves by caterpillars is beneficial to the plant's growth and development. It was found that damaged radish leaves produced chemicals that protected the plant from attack by other destructive insects, and that the damaged radish plants produced more seed than undamaged plants[7]. This phenomenon can also be seen in the agricultural practice of pinching shoots off fruit trees every spring, or peeling a piece of bark from the trunk, in order to obtain a good harvest in the fall. In the case of human beings, the minimal trauma caused by needling can relieve the maximal suffering caused by illness. This example of the Law of Paradox or Contradiction leads us to predict that although new acupuncture techniques and new methods of stimulating the acupoints may be developed, needling will always remain primary in the clinical practice of acupuncture.

It is clear that during acupuncture treatment the doctor, the needle and the patient form an integrated cycle. The doctor manipulates the needle, the needle traumatizes the patient's body and arouses the self-healing force, and the self-healing force works to automatically harmonize the imbalance. If the cycle is incomplete, the treatment is likely to be ineffective. Acupuncture is therefore holistic in its practice, as well as in its underlying theory. In the cycle of treatment and healing, the self-healing force within the patient's body is primary, the needling stimulation is secondary, and the needle establishes a bridge between the patient and doctor.

Needling methods

Following identification of the pattern of a disorder in the clinic, appropriate needling methods are selected according to its nature. The two basic needling methods, reducing and reinforcing, are used for excessive and deficient conditions respectively.

It must be pointed out that the terms 'reducing' or 'reinforcing' refer to the results of treatment, rather than the process itself. Because acupuncture treats disease by arousing and strengthening the body's self-healing force, it could be considered that needling is always reinforcing, no matter which needling method is used. Take bacterial dysentery, for example. According to traditional Chinese medicine, bacterial dysentery is an excessive damp-heat condition. Treatment consists of applying reducing manipulation, or even bloodletting puncturing, in order to dispel damp and cool heat. Although this treatment has a reducing effect, it works by reinforcing the body's self-healing force, or right *qi*.

Another common misunderstanding about needling is that forceful needling manipulation has a reducing effect and mild needling manipulation has a reinforcing effect. The fact is that, thanks to the bi-directional effect, needling the same acupoint with the same method may produce opposite effects under different circumstances. That is, there will be a reinforcing effect if the condition is deficient, while there will be a reducing effect if the condition is excessive. The results of acupuncture are primarily determined by the patient's condition. The body's self-healing force tends to harmonize the condition automatically, by reducing excess or reinforcing deficiency as the case demands.

Needling can be compared to shooting a crossbow. If the trigger can be correctly located, very mild stimulation will produce a great effect. The *Neijing* states: 'Experts won't lightly load the bow, for fear of accidental firing; whereas the inexpert can't fire the bow, no matter how they flail'[8].

Of course needling will not always produce a balancing effect, especially in the case of extreme conditions. If reducing manipulation is applied to an extremely deficient condition, there may be profuse sweating, dizziness, pale complexion, or even loss of consciousness. This is like kicking a person who is already down. Conversely, if reinforcing manipulation is applied to an extremely excessive condition, the condition will also take a turn for the worse. This is like using oil to try to put out a bonfire.

Therefore, although the body is endowed with self-healing properties, treatment must still utilize the appropriate method of stimulation if satisfactory results are to be achieved. The *Neijing* warns: 'The condition may become worse if one applies the reducing method to a deficiency or vice versa'[9].

Eight needling methods are commonly used in clinical practice. Their manipulations and applications are as follows.

Table 4.1
Reducing and reinforcing needling manipulations

Manipulation	Reducing	Reinforcing
Lifting–thrusting	Insert the needle to a given depth. Alternately lift forcefully and rapidly, and thrust gently and slowly	Insert the needle to a given depth. Alternately lift gently and slowly, and thrust forcefully and rapidly
Rotating	Insert the needle to a given depth. Rotate rapidly and forcefully in large circles	Insert the needle to a given depth. Rotate gently and slowly in small circles
Breathing	Insert the needle on the patient's exhale and withdraw on the inhale	Insert the needle on the patient's inhale and withdraw on the exhale
Directional	Insert the needle slanted against the course of the meridian	Insert needle slanted along the course of the meridian
Fast–slow	Insert the needle rapidly and withdraw slowly	Insert the needle slowly and withdraw rapidly
Opening and closing	Shake the needle while withdrawing in order to enlarge the hole and allow pathogens to escape	Press the needled area while withdrawing in order to close the hole and prevent right *qi* from escaping

Reducing method

The reducing method is one of the two basic types of needling stimulation. It is used to expel pathogens and in the case of excessive conditions. There are a number of needling variations, which may be applied either singly or in combination. (See Table 4.1.) These include lifting–thrusting and rotating manipulation, the most frequently used, and bloodletting puncturing, used to reduce heat pathogens in the case of excessive heat conditions. Moxibustion is usually combined with reducing needling in the case of excessive cold conditions.

Reinforcing method

The reinforcing method is the second of the two basic types of needling stimulation. It is used to supplement deficiency of right *qi*, and in the case of deficient conditions. There are a number of needling variations, which may be applied either singly or in combination. (See Table 4.1.) Moxibustion may be combined with reinforcing needling, except in cases of yin deficiency. It should be noted that if the condition is extremely deficient, it is better not to use acupuncture, but rather to choose other therapies. The *Neijing* suggests: 'If there is deficiency of both yin and yang *qi*, apply sweet herbs [which have tonifying properties] instead of acupuncture'[10].

Cooling method

The reducing needling manipulations described above and bloodletting puncturing are used to cool heat in excessive heat conditions. In addition, a comprehensive cooling method called 'Cooling the Sky', first recorded in the *Ode of Golden Needles*, may be used in either excessive or deficient heat conditions[11].

'Cooling the Sky' divides the acupoint into three layers, superficial, middle and deep, corresponding to Sky, Human and Earth respectively. The needle is quickly inserted to the

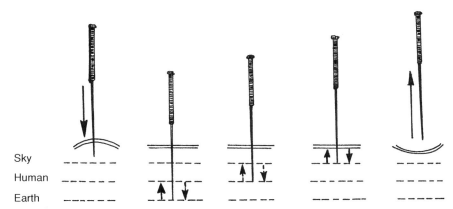

Sky

Human

Earth

Figure 4.1   'Cooling the Sky' needling manipulation.

deep layer, and either lifted forcefully and rapidly and thrust lightly and slowly, or rotated quickly in large circles, six times at this depth. The needle is then withdrawn to the middle layer and the manipulation repeated, and finally withdrawn to the superficial layer and the manipulation repeated. The entire process should be repeated several times, until the patient experiences a cool feeling in the needled area or even throughout the whole body in some cases. The needle is not withdrawn and reinserted between layers, but rather stays in the body during the entire process. Finally, the needle is slowly withdrawn completely as the patient exhales, and the hole is kept open. (See Figure 4.1.)

Warming method

Either reducing or reinforcing manipulation is used to warm cold, depending on whether the condition is excessive or deficient. Moxibustion or cupping may be used in combination with reducing needling in excessive conditions, and moxibustion or cupping may be used in combination with reinforcing needling in deficient conditions. In addition, a comprehensive warming method called 'Firing the Mountain', first recorded in the *Ode of Golden Needles*, may be used in either excessive or deficient cold conditions[12].

The manipulation used in 'Firing the Mountain' is opposite to that of 'Cooling the Sky'. The needle is slowly inserted to the superficial layer, and either thrust forcefully and rapidly and lifted lightly and slowly, or rotated slowly in small circles, nine times at this depth. The needle is then inserted to the middle layer and the manipulation repeated, and finally inserted to the deep layer and the manipulation repeated. The entire process should be repeated several times until the patient experiences a warm feeling in the needled area, or even throughout the whole body in some cases. The needle is not withdrawn and reinserted between layers, but rather stays in the body during the entire process. Finally, the needle is quickly withdrawn completely as the patient inhales, and the hole is pressed closed. (See Figure 4.2.)

Sweating method

The sweating method is a variation of the reducing method used to induce perspiration and expel exterior pathogens. The *Neijing* states: 'Induce sweating to expel pathogens when

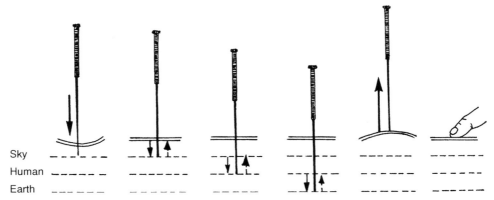

Figure 4.2 'Firing the Mountain' needling manipulation.

they are within the skin'[13]. The sweating method is applied primarily to two conditions in clinical practice:

1. It is used to expel wind-cold in cases of excessive wind-cold type common cold or influenza. This condition is marked by chills, no sweating, headache, general achiness, dilute nasal discharge or obstruction, a thin white tongue coating, and a superficial tense pulse. Commonly used acupoints include LI4-Hegu, GB20-Fengchi, DU14-Dazhui and UB13-Feishu. 'Firing the Mountain' is used to induce a hot needling sensation and cause sweating; moxibustion or cupping may also be added.
2. It is used to clear heat in cases of excessive wind-heat type common cold or influenza. This condition is marked by fever, headache, sore throat, thirst, cough with yellow sputum, a red tongue tip with a thin yellow coating, and a superficial, forceful, rapid pulse. Commonly used acupoints include DU14-Dazhui, UB13-Feishu, LU6-Kongzui and LU11-Shaoshang. 'Cooling the Sky' is used to induce a cool needling sensation and cause sweating; bloodletting puncturing and cupping may also be added.

Ejection method

The ejection method is a variation of the reducing method used to expel pathogens from the Upper or Middle Jiao upward through the mouth. The *Neijing* states: 'Eject pathogens when they are higher in the body'[14]. The ejection method is applied primarily to two conditions in clinical practice:

1. Expectoration is induced to eject turbid phlegm that is obstructing the Upper Jiao. This condition is marked by a feeling of fullness in the chest, shortness of breath, non-productive cough, and rattling phlegm in the throat; or sudden loss of consciousness with foaming at the mouth. RN22-Tiantu is pressed with the thumb of the left hand until the patient feels the urge to cough. This point is then quickly punctured to cause the patient to expectorate the turbid phlegm. If there is no ejection of phlegm, Ex-Jialianquan (about 1 *cun* bilateral to RN23-Lianquan) can be added to increase stimulation.
2. Vomiting is induced to eject retained food or toxins from the stomach that are obstructing the Middle Jiao. This condition is marked by severe distension or pain in the epigastric region, nausea with inability to vomit, and even loss of consciousness.

The patient usually has a history of intake of toxins or overeating food that is difficult to digest. PC6-Neiguan is punctured using the reducing method to induce vomiting. If this is not effective, RN12-Zhongwan can be added to increase stimulation.

Purging method

The purging method is used to expel pathogens from the Lower Jiao downward through the bowels. This method may be either reducing or reinforcing, depending on whether the condition is excessive or deficient. The *Neijing* states: 'Purge pathogens when they are lower in the body'[15].

Constipation is a typical example of pathogens obstructing the Lower Jiao. This condition is generally divided into excessive and deficient types. Excessive constipation is usually due to excessive heat consuming the yin fluids. It is marked by constipation, abdominal pain aggravated by pressure, a red or purple tongue with a thick, dry, yellow coating, and a forceful rapid pulse. Acupoints used for this condition include ST25-Tianshu, ST37-Shangjuxu, ST44-Neiting and SJ6-Zhigou. The reducing method is applied to cool heat and loosen the bowel. This method is also known as 'raking the firewood from beneath the cauldron'.

Deficient constipation may be caused by an insufficiency of *qi* and blood to moisten the bowels, as in the case of the elderly or postpartum women. There may be no manifestation other than constipation. Acupoints used to treat this condition include ST25-Tianshu, ST36-Zusanli, UB25-Dachangshu, SP6-Sanyinjiao and SP15-Daheng. Either the even method (see below) or the reinforcing method is applied to nourish the body fluid and move the hard stool. This method is also known as 'increasing fluid to refloat the grounded ship'.

Another example of pathogens obstructing the Lower Jiao is dysentery due to accumulation of damp-heat in the bowels. This condition is marked by abdominal pain, diarrhea with pus and blood, abdominal urgency and rectal heaviness (tenesmus), a red tongue with a sticky yellow coating, and a slippery rapid pulse. Acupoints used to treat this condition include ST25-Tianshu, ST29-Guilai, RN3-Zhongji, SP9-Yinlingquan, ST44-Neiting and LI4-Hegu. The reducing method is applied to cool heat and drain dampness.

Harmonizing or even method

The harmonizing method, popularly known as the even method, falls between the reducing and reinforcing methods. The needle is either lifted and thrust, or rotated, evenly and gently at moderate speed, and is withdrawn at moderate speed. The even method is applied primarily to two conditions in clinical practice:

1. It is used to harmonize the Gallbladder Meridian of Foot Shaoyang. This meridian is located on the bilateral sides of the body, between the Stomach Meridian of Foot Yangming in the front and the Urinary Bladder of Foot Taiyang on the back. Since the Urinary Bladder Meridian is considered to be exterior and the Stomach Meridian interior, the Gallbladder Meridian is considered to be half interior and half exterior. When pathogens invade the half interior-half exterior Gallbladder Meridian of Foot Shaoyang, there will be a bitter taste in the mouth, dry throat, blurred vision, alternating chills and fever, a feeling of fullness in the chest, poor appetite, vomiting, and silence or restlessness. This condition is called Shaoyang Pattern. Shaoyang Pattern is common to many diseases, including the common cold, influenza, gallstones,

cholecystitis and malaria. In many cases, only one or several typical manifestations of Shaoyang Pattern may be present. For example, some cases are marked by a bitter taste in the mouth and alternating chills and fever, while others are marked by vomiting and depression. The Chinese medical sage Zhang Zhongjing, a noted practitioner of the Eastern Han Dynasty (25–220 AD), states in the *Discussion of Cold-Induced Diseases* (*Shanghan Lun*): 'In cases of cold-induced conditions, it is Shaoyang Pattern even if only one manifestation of the pattern appears'[16]. When treating Shaoyang Pattern, it is forbidden to use either the sweating method (which should be reserved for exterior heat or cold conditions) or the purging method (which is reserved for excessive interior heat conditions). Only the even needling method should be applied to harmonize the Shaoyang Meridian. The main acupoints used for Shaoyang Pattern include GB20-Fengchi, GB34-Yanglingquan and PC6-Neiguan.

2. It is used to harmonize conditions that show no obvious manifestations of either excess or deficiency. When it is difficult to identify the nature of a condition, the even method, midway between the reducing and reinforcing methods, should be chosen.

Enhancing the needling sensation

Achievement of the needling sensation is the sole standard by which to judge if acupuncture will be effective in either excessive/deficient or heat/cold conditions. The stronger the needling sensation and the more quickly it is obtained, the better the results will be and the faster the cure. Therefore, the main purpose of acupuncture is to induce and maximize the needling sensation, regardless of which needling method is used.

Many factors may influence the strength of the needling sensation, including individual differences, the nature of the illness, the strength of the patient's self-healing force, the temperature of the environment, the accuracy with which acupoints are selected and located, the needling method, and even the mood of both patient and practitioner. All of these factors should be taken into consideration in order to maximize the needling sensation.

Acupuncture treatment should be carried out in three stages: preparation, manipulation and retention.

Stage one: preparation

Palpating the acupoints to be needled
Palpating the acupoints to be needled has two purposes. First, as mentioned in Chapters 2 and 3, palpating allows the practitioner accurately to locate the acupoints to be treated. When disease or disorder is present, positive reactions such as tenderness and bumps will often manifest on or near acupoints of the affected meridians. A good needling sensation will be obtained if (and only if) needling is applied exactly at the location of the positive reactions. Although positive reactions may occur precisely at the theoretical locations of the acupoints, often they are slightly removed. It is therefore necessary to determine the exact location of the positive points by means of palpation. The *Neijing* recommends first pressing the acupoint, and puncturing it only if the patient feels tenderness or the pain is relieved[17]. This is particularly important when puncturing specific acupoints such as back *shu* (transport) acupoints, front *mu* (assembly) acupoints and *he* (sea) acupoints.

Secondly, palpating the acupoints can activate the local flow of *qi* and blood. This will cause the patient to feel less pain when the needles are inserted, and will also make it easier to induce arrival of *qi*.

Pressing, tapping or massaging along the pathways of the affected meridians
The main purpose of this action is to activate the flow of *qi* and blood in the affected
meridians so that the needling sensation can be more easily induced. The *Compendium of
Acupuncture and Moxibustion* states: 'Press up and down the course of the affected
meridian to promote the flow of *qi* and blood'[18]. This is especially important when
treating deficient conditions, since in these cases the patient's right *qi* is deficient and
arrival of *qi* is usually slow and weak, sometimes not occurring until well into the
treatment. The *Neijing* suggests pressing both the acupoints and the meridians before
needling in cases of deficiency[19].

Warming the affected meridians (except in excessive heat conditions)
Apply moxibustion or any other means to warm the affected meridians before puncturing.
Just as water flows freely when the weather is warm, so warming the pathways of the
meridians can promote transmission of the needling sensation. (See Chapter 2 for
discussion of the role of warmth in meridian transmission.) The clinic should be kept
warm (preferably above 26°C). Warming the meridians is especially advisable for cold
conditions, either excessive or deficient, but is forbidden for excessive heat conditions.

Warming the needles before puncturing
The practice of warming the needles prior to puncturing has a long history. The
Compendium of Acupuncture and Moxibustion, written in 1601 AD toward the end of the
Ming Dynasty (1368–1644 AD), states: 'Before puncturing, put the needles in your mouth
or close to your body to warm them, so that it will be easy to promote the flow of *qi* and
blood. It is also suitable to warm needles in boiling water'[20]. The method of warming
needles in the mouth was discarded long ago, but this record is a reminder that warming
the needles is an effective way to increase the needling sensation. At the very least,
puncturing with cold needles should be avoided.

Stage two: manipulation

Manipulating the needles is the most important step in inducing the needling sensation. In
addition to the subjective perception of the needling sensation experienced by the patient,
manifestations will also be felt by the practitioner. When *qi* arrives, the needle will feel
heavy in the practitioner's hand and will resist rotation or lifting–thrusting, as described
in the *Lyrics of Standard Profundities*: 'If the needle feels light and loose, *qi* has not yet
arrived; but if the needle is heavy and tense, *qi* is coming'[21]. Therefore, in addition to
inquiring about and observing the patient's reactions during manipulation, the practitioner
should concentrate the mind on the hand that is manipulating the needles in order to judge
whether or not the needling sensation has been achieved.

   In general, the duration of the manipulating stage depends upon when the needling
sensation is achieved. The *Neijing* suggests: 'Manipulate the needle without stopping until
there is arrival of *qi*; stop manipulating when *qi* arrives'[22]. Of course, this does not mean
that one should manipulate the needle endlessly if there is no arrival of *qi*. If the needling
sensation has not been obtained after several minutes of manipulation, the following
factors should be considered before proceeding.

Location of acupoints and angle or depth of insertion of the needle
The needling sensation will be achieved only if the correct acupoints are punctured. If
there is no needling sensation because the acupoints have been inaccurately located or the
needle has been inserted at the wrong angle or improper depth, the needle should be

withdrawn and reinserted at the correct location, or the angle and depth of the needle adjusted.

Individual differences

Every person responds differently to needling stimulation, and this human factor plays an important role in acupuncture treatment. Some people are very sensitive to needling stimulation and experience the needling sensation quickly and strongly, indicating that there will be good therapeutic results. Others are relatively insensitive to needling stimulation and experience the needling sensation slowly and weakly, or not at all, no matter what kind of manipulation is applied. In the latter case, if there has been no improvement in the condition after one course of treatment (usually five sessions) the practitioner should recommend treatment with therapies other than acupuncture.

Additionally, a patient's experience of the needling sensation may vary when the same acupoint is punctured by different practitioners. This phenomenon may be related to differences in the practitioners' innate qualities, as well as in their technical ability. An essay in the *Neijing* entitled 'Appoint occupations according to ability' states that people selected for training in acupuncture and moxibustion should be soft-spoken, contained, skillful and attentive[23].

Nature of the condition

The strength of the needling sensation is influenced by the nature of the condition. In excessive and heat conditions, arrival of *qi* is usually quick and strong, while in cold and deficient conditions, arrival of *qi* is usually slow and weak, and in some cases does not occur until well into the treatment. In cases of slow or weak arrival of *qi*, additional preparatory stimulation should be applied to the meridians, and additional auxiliary manipulation applied to the needles during the retention stage. As the patient's condition improves, the needling sensation may be more easily achieved and become progressively stronger.

In some extremely severe excessive or deficient conditions, arrival of *qi* may never occur. This is a bad sign, and indicates that the patient's self-healing force is severely depleted.

Stage three: retention

After the manipulating stage, the needles are usually retained within the body for a period of time rather than withdrawn immediately. There are three reasons to retain the needles: to maintain the needling sensation, to promote the needling sensation, and to await the arrival of *qi*.

Maintaining the needling sensation

A strong needling sensation will sometimes persist following completion of the basic needling manipulation. The patient may experience extreme soreness and distension in the needled region, and in some cases may report a sensation that the needle is intermittently thrusting by itself. This phenomenon is described in the *Lyrics of Standard Profundities* as follows: 'When *qi* arrives, the patient will have the internal sensation that the needle is moving up and down, much like the movement of a fishing line float after a fish has been hooked'[24].

Upon arrival of *qi*, the practitioner may feel that the needle is tense and have difficulty manipulating it. This usually occurs in excessive conditions or in patients who are very sensitive to needling stimulation. If such a strong needling sensation occurs, the needles should be retained until the needling sensation decreases. The *Ode of Golden Needles* states[25]:

> If the condition is not alleviated after needling, the needles will be like something rooted in the body and cannot be twirled or thrust. This indicates that the evil *qi* is sucking the needles and the right *qi* has not yet arrived. When this occurs, retain the needle and withdraw it only when it becomes loose.

Promoting the needling sensation

If the patient experiences only mild or moderate soreness and distension in the needled area following completion of the basic needling manipulation, and the practitioner can thrust or rotate the needles easily, further measures may be taken to increase the flow of *qi* and blood and promote the needling sensation. In addition to repeating the preparatory measures and basic needling manipulation at intervals, the following auxiliary manipulating methods can be applied during the retention stage:

- *Snapping.* Snap the handle of the needle lightly to make the needle tremble slightly. (See Figure 4.3.)
- *Scraping.* Keeping the thumb of the right hand on the handle of the needle to hold it steady, scrape up and down the handle with the nail of the index or middle finger of the right hand. (See Figure 4.4.)
- *Shaking.* Shake the handle or body of the needle lightly. (See Figure 4.5.)
- *Twisting.* Twist the needle clockwise with the thumb and index finger and then separate the fingers quickly. Repeat the manipulation several times. Because this manipulation resembles a flying bird, it is also called 'flying needling'. (See Figure 4.6.)
- *Vibrating.* Hold the needle with the fingers of the right hand and apply small, quick, lifting–thrusting movements to cause vibration.

These auxiliary manipulating methods can be used either singly or in combination with the basic needling methods.

Waiting for arrival of qi

If following basic manipulation there is no needling sensation, and all possibilities that may have prevented the needling sensation from being achieved have been ruled out, the

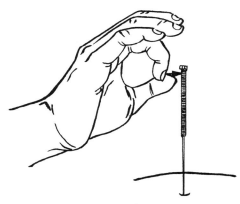

Figure 4.3   Supplementary needling manipulation: snapping.

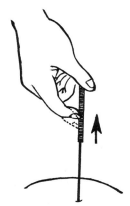

Figure 4.4 Supplementary needling manipulation: scraping.

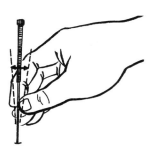

Figure 4.5 Supplementary needling manipulation: shaking.

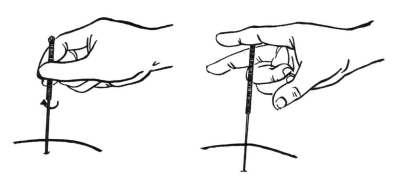

Figure 4.6 Supplementary needling manipulation: twisting.

needles should be retained while patient and practitioner concentrate their minds and patiently wait for arrival of *qi*. The *Neijing* suggests: 'Wait very attentively until *qi* arrives. It is like awaiting a distinguished guest; do not heed the setting sun'[26].

The needles can generally be retained for 15–30 minutes at this stage. While retaining the needles, the methods suggested for promoting the needling sensation during the preparatory and manipulating stages may be repeated at intervals.

For some chronic and refractory conditions, long-term retention of the needles is necessary: 6 hours, 12 hours, or even more. One practitioner reported treating a case of tetanus with acupuncture. The tetanus stopped after each insertion of the needles, but recurred as soon as the needles were removed. He finally retained the needles for 48 hours and the patient was cured[27].

Mental concentration

Finally, the importance of mental concentration by both practitioner and patient cannot be overemphasized. Acupuncture is not a purely physical therapy. The power of the will, unique to human beings, is important to the healing process. In *qigong*, the practice of the mental control of *qi*, *qi* can be directed along the meridians by will alone. *Qi* may arrive quickly and strongly if acupuncture treatment is supported by the mind's ability to control the flow of *qi*. The patient should cultivate positive belief and confidence in the efficacy of the treatment, while concentrating the mind to lead *qi* to the affected area.

The *Neijing* states[28]:

> The key to acupuncture is first of all to *zhi shen* 治神 – concentrate the spirit. Regardless of how deep or shallow the acupoint, or whether it is distal or proximal, when needling you must focus your spirit as if facing an abyss one thousand feet deep. Everything must be done with delicate care. When manipulating the needles with your fingertips, you should handle the needles as if handling a fierce tiger. Focus all your attention.

A quiet and comfortable environment will help both patient and practitioner to concentrate their minds better.

Indications and contraindications of acupuncture

People tend to go to extremes when considering the proper scope of acupuncture. Some think the use of acupuncture should be very limited. They apply it only for a few conditions, such as pain and motor impairment. Others inflate its applications, and consider acupuncture to be a panacea. Both extremes are incorrect. In fact, once the theory behind acupuncture treatment is fully grasped, its indications and contraindications become clear.

Indications

Inflammatory conditions
Inflammation is the body's normal defense reaction to local injury, infection, necrosis, allergy or other local irritation. It is one of the most important self-healing mechanisms within the body. When the body is injured, the self-healing force will try to deal with the injury and repair itself. If the self-healing force is strong and eventually defeats the injury, there will be a cure. Otherwise, the condition will persist or even spread.

inflammation is generally a desirable reaction, it is better to promote the
ry response and speed up its successful resolution rather than try to suppress
ture treats inflammation by mobilizing the body's self-healing force so that it
ɘ body to deal effectively with the injury. Experiments show that acupuncture
has powerful effects on the inflammatory response. It can regulate the local inflammatory
process, control the inflammatory reaction, shorten the inflammatory process, regulate
proliferation of granulation tissue and decrease adhesion after surgery. Moreover, it
influences specific and non-specific cellular and humoral immunity[29].

Although inflammation is generally a positive self-healing mechanism, it may
sometimes create problems when it occurs in response to allergens that gain entry to the
body through inhalation, ingestion or skin contact. Because of its bi-directional beneficial
effect, acupuncture can suppress inflammation that occurs due to allergy.

Acupuncture is a highly effective means of treating clinical inflammatory conditions,
especially microbial infections. There has been great improvement in the treatment of
infection since the discovery of penicillin in the 1930s. However, acupuncture has several
major advantages over drugs in the treatment of microbial problems:

1. Acupuncture has no side effects. Drugs kill microbes directly, and are valuable when
   used appropriately; however, incorrect or excessive use of antimicrobial drugs can
   result in a variety of side effects, some severe, such as damage to the immune system,
   destruction of the body's beneficial flora, and breeding of resistant strains of bacteria.
   Acupuncture, by contrast, mobilizes the body's innate self-healing force, which
   operates by selectively killing only harmful (and not beneficial) microorganisms.
   During this process, the body's immune system is strengthened rather than damaged,
   harmful bacteria do not develop resistance, and balance is restored among the flora that
   inhabit the body.
2. Acupuncture is broad-spectrum. Drugs are effective mainly against specific types of
   bacteria and some parasites. However, more resistant and dangerous strains of bacteria
   are appearing all the time. Also, despite the progress made in drug therapy since the
   onset of the AIDS crisis, there are still no satisfactory antivirals. Acupuncture, on the
   other hand, strengthens the overall self-healing force and increases the body's innate
   ability to recognize and kill most disease-causing microbes, including viruses, bacteria,
   fungi and some protozoa.
3. Acupuncture simultaneously treats both Root and Tip. According to the principle of
   Root and Tip, in cases of infection the body's self-healing force is the Root and the
   microbes are the Tip. Drugs, by killing the microbes, treat only the Tip. Acupuncture
   activates the body's self-healing force to treat the Root of the condition. Additionally,
   acupuncture relieves many symptoms of infectious diseases such as fever and pain,
   which are the Tip of the disease. Therefore, acupuncture treats both the Root and Tip
   of infections simultaneously.

Pain conditions

Pain is a symptom of many diseases. Although pain is almost synonymous with suffering,
it also has great significance in self-preservation. Pain is a signal that something harmful
is invading the body, either internally or externally. If people feel no pain when their
bodies come under attack, they will fail to defend themselves and will suffer injury.
Therefore, while the factors that lead to pain are our enemies, pain itself is our friend.

Take coronary heart disease, for example. Although some people with heart disease
suffer only mild pathological changes, they experience substantial pain and are therefore
spurred to adopt measures to prevent the situation from deteriorating. On the other hand,

some people may have severe pathological changes accompanied by little or no pain, so they become careless and may suffer a sudden attack of cardiac infarction.

We often fail to recognize pain as beneficial in daily life. Patients and doctors alike are often gripped by the suffering caused by pain, while neglecting its significance. Everyone tries to suppress pain. Many painkillers have been invented for this purpose. Such drugs function mainly to mask the pain, while leaving its cause untouched. Consequently, patients often become trapped in a cycle of dependency on the continuous intake of drugs. If administration of painkillers does not work, they may attempt the last resort of blocking or even severing the nerves that transmit the pain signal. All of these methods are no better than burying one's head in the sand, or plugging one's ears while stealing a bell. They do nothing to deal with the root of the problem.

Acupuncture, on the other hand, mobilizes the body's own self-healing force to deal with pain. As discussed in Chapter 1, filiform needling, the most typical and common type of acupuncture used today, was originally devised to treat *bi* syndrome or joint pain, one of the most commonly seen pain conditions. Pain relief is one of the oldest, most well-known and widely used applications of acupuncture. New developments in this area include the use of acupuncture for anesthesia during surgery since the 1950s[30]. Acupuncture has typically first been recognized in countries outside of China for its effectiveness in pain relief, and it is now used for a wide range of pain conditions throughout the world.

Needling the body causes pain, but it can relieve pre-existing pain. What is the mechanism behind this contradiction? One theory of acupuncture anesthesia suggests that insertion of acupuncture needles may stimulate the release of endorphins, a type of natural opiate analog produced within the brain. These substances are remarkably potent painkillers, and could be responsible for dulling the pain impulses caused by surgical procedures[31].

The release of endorphins by acupuncture may be only part of its pain-relieving mechanism. The action of naturally produced endorphins in suppressing pain is similar to that of painkillers, with the difference that the former are endogenous while the latter are exogenous. More important, however, is the fact that acupuncture treats the causes of which pain is a symptom. For instance, acupuncture relieves smooth muscle spasm, thereby greatly reducing pain in conditions such as gastric spasm; biliary, renal, uterine and gastrointestinal colic; peripheral circulatory upset; and asthma. Acupuncture functions both to suppress the feeling of pain and to cut off its cause, treating both Root and Tip, indicating that it is an optimal method for treating pain.

Physical and mental dysfunction
Physical and mental dysfunction account for most diseases and disorders seen in clinical practice. Such disorders are due to physiological imbalance, and are accompanied by no obvious organic changes. They are a result of the body's failure to regulate itself and adapt to change, and subsequent hyperfunction or hypofunction of various systems.

Acupuncture can effectively assist the body's self-regulating ability, so that hyperfunction will be inhibited while hypofunction is excited. Acupuncture can harmonize almost all dysfunctions, psychological and physiological, somatic and autonomic. For instance, acupuncture is very effective for a variety of functional problems of the gastrointestinal tract, including esophagospasm, vomiting, gastric spasm, gastroatoma, anorexia, enterospasm, flatulence, irritable bowel syndrome, constipation and gastro-intestinal neurosis.

Another advantage of acupuncture lies in its method of treatment. Medications, both modern drugs and traditional herbs, have unidirectional effects. This means that a medication is either inhibitory or excitatory, but never both. Accordingly, inappropriate use of medications, such as the application of inhibitory drugs for a depressive condition or stimulants for an excitatory condition, will worsen the condition. Furthermore, abuse of drugs may lead to over-inhibition or over-stimulation. For instance, patients who abuse sedatives may experience dizziness, lassitude, distractibility and even addiction. Finally, there are still no satisfactory drugs for a number of dysfunctions, such as depression, anorexia and gastrointestinal weakness. However, acupuncture can assist the body to harmonize the dysfunction precisely, whether it is a case of hypofunction or hyperfunction.

Acupuncture is indicated for the following conditions:

- Infectious diseases – typhoid, paratyphoid, cholera, bacterial dysentery, brucellosis, venereal disease, tuberculosis, mumps, viral B encephalitis, viral hepatitis, the common cold, influenza, herpes zoster, malaria, schistosomiasis, filariasis, amebic dysentery, tinea pedis.
- Neurological disorders – headache, migraine, epilepsy, tetanus, sequelae of cerebrovascular accident such as hemiplegia and aphasia, facial nerve spasms or paralysis, trigeminal and intercostal neuralgia, sciatica, peripheral neuropathy.
- Emotional and psychological disorders – anxiety, depression, excitability, worry, fearful states, schizophrenia, manic-depressive psychosis, involutional psychosis, reactive psychosis, neurasthenia, anxiety state, phobic state, hysteria, obsessive–compulsive neurosis.
- Gastrointestinal disorders – stomatitis, gingivitis, glossitis, globus hystericus, polysalia, esophagospasm, esophagitis, cardiospasm, pylorospasm, hiccups, hyperhydrochloria, hypohydrochloria, air-swallowing (erophagia), gastrospasm, gastric dilatation, volvulus of the stomach, gastric ptosis, peptic ulcer, anorexia, indigestion, gastrointestinal weakness, gastritis, duodenitis, enteritis, food allergies, food poisoning, gastrointestinal neurosis, acute simple or chronic appendicitis, irritable bowel syndrome, enterospasm, twisting of the bowel, spastic or paralytic ileus, constipation, prolapse of the anus, hemorrhoids, chronic pancreatitis, cholecystitis, gallstones, hepatitis.
- Respiratory diseases – tonsillitis, pharyngitis, laryngitis, tracheitis, bronchitis, bronchial asthma, bronchiectasis, pneumonia.
- Genitourinary problems – nephritis, cystitis, urethritis, incontinence or retention of urine, nervous frequent urination, urinary stones, prostatitis, prostatic hyperplasia, testitis, hydrocele testis, sexual dysfunction, impotence, priapism, seminal emission, premature ejaculation, infertility.
- Circulatory disorders – hypertension, hypotension, arrhythmia, cardiac neurosis, coronary heart disease, myocarditis, endocarditis, pulseless disease, erythromelalgia, Raynaud's disease, anemia.
- Diseases of the sensory organs – otitis, nervous tinnitus or deafness, toxic deafness, epistaxis, rhinitis, sinusitis; styes, night blindness, retinitis, optic atrophy, conjunctivitis, keratitis, glaucoma.
- Cutaneous and subcutaneous diseases – urticaria, eczema, pruritus, carbuncle, furunculosis, neurodermatitis, hyperhidrosis, hypohidrosis, acne.
- Infantile problems – pertussis, diphtheria, indigestion, malnutrition, constipation, infantile paralysis, infantile convulsions, chorea rheumatica, minimal brain dysfunction syndrome (MBD), mental retardation, night crying, sleepwalking, nocturnal enuresis, infantile psychoses, myogenic torticollis, myopia, strabismus, inguinal hernia.

- Gynecological disorders – dysmenorrhea, pre
  amenorrhea, menopausal syndrome, morning sick
  difficult labor, prolapsed uterus, mastitis, fibrocy
- Musculoskeletal problems – arthritis, frozen shoulde,
  spondylosis, lower back pain, sprains, strains, tendoniu.
- Emergency – high fever, shock, convulsions, loss of cᴜ
  drowning, poisoning.
- Others – addictions such as alcohol, nicotine and drugs; treatment o
  effects from general anesthesia, parturition, surgery, cytotoxic cheɪ.
  ionizing radiation.

Contraindications

Damaged self-healing system

Acupuncture in itself is nothing. It works through the body's self-healing force, which is related to the functions of the nerves, the endocrine glands and the immune system, as well as functions that may still be unknown. Therefore, from the treatment point of view, acupuncture will work well when the body's self-healing system is intact, but it will be useless if this system has been compromised by either congenital or acquired factors. For example, acupuncture is very effective for nocturnal enuresis due to functional disturbance, but it is ineffective for cases caused by congenital spina bifida; it is very effective for infectious diseases, but it is of no use if the patient has immunological problems.

Irreversible organic problems

Acupuncture can assist damaged tissue to recover, if tissue regeneration is possible. For instance, the skin and liver have marked regenerative capacities. Acupuncture can stimulate regeneration of these tissues by improving local circulation and countering inflammation and infection. However, it cannot stimulate recovery of tissues that are incapable of regenerating, such as in cases of spinal cord injury, brain damage, perforation due to gastric ulcer, prolapse of intervertebral discs, and many types of tumors. There will be no benefit from acupuncture treatment in such cases, even if the patient's self-healing system is intact. For example, acupuncture can lower the level of blood sugar in cases of insulin-independent diabetes (type II diabetes), but it is of no use in cases of insulin-dependent diabetes (type I diabetes). It can effectively relieve headaches due to functional disturbance, but is of no use for headaches due to tumors, either benign or malignant, within the skull. In these cases other therapies are required.

Extremely deficient conditions

The fundamental prerequisite for the successful application of acupuncture is that the natural healing force be present within the body. Although acupuncture can strengthen the body's self-healing force to treat deficient conditions, needling will not be effective if the self-healing force is extremely deficient. On the contrary, acupuncture may damage the self-healing force even further, especially if the reducing needling method is applied. The *Neijing* states[32]:

> Do not treat with needles if both yin and yang *qi* are deficient. Treating such a condition with needles will increase the deficiency. The body's blood and yin and yang *qi* will be exhausted, the five *zang* organs will become vacant, and the tendons, bones, and marrow will dry up. Consequently, the aged will die and adults will not recover.

Such cases should rather be treated with tonifying herbs[33].

fection, acupuncture indirectly helps to kill microbes (the Tip) by
the immune functions (the Root). However, if the infection is severe and the
are extremely strong, antimicrobials should be given first to treat the Tip. In
practice, acupuncture can be used in combination with antimicrobials in order to
ease their side effects.

Notes and References

1. Tang De'an *et al.*, *Experimental Acupuncture and Moxibustion* (*Shiyan Zhenjiu Xue* 实验针灸学). Tianjin: Publishing House of Tianjin College of Traditional Chinese Medicine, 1983, pp. 81–83.
2. *Suwen*, 72:581.
3. Louis Pasteur (1822–1895), the founder of microbiology, apparently recognized this fact as significant. On his deathbed, the great scientist is said to have told friends that his archrival, Claude Bernard, was correct in maintaining that the body withstands disease or embraces it by virtue of its overall health. 'Bernard is right,' Pasteur confided. 'Microbes are nothing, the soil is everything.' From Tom Monte *et al.*, *World Medicine – The East–West Guide to Healing Your Body*, p. 56.
4. *Suwen*, 33:197.
5. *Lingshu*, 1:3.
6. *The Ode of Golden Needles* (*Jinzhen Fu* 金针赋), quoted in Xu Feng, *The Complete Book of Acupuncture and Moxibustion* (*Zhenjiu Daquan* 针灸大全) (1439 AD). Beijing: People's Health Press, 1987, p. 123. *The Ode of Golden Needles* was written by an unnamed hermit during the Ming Dynasty (1368–1644 AD). It is the most influential work on needling manipulation in the history of acupuncture, and the source of most manipulating methods in use today.
7. *Beijing Evening News* (*Beijing Wanbao* 北京晚报), March 12, 1998, p. 16.
8. *Lingshu*, 1:1.
9. *Ibid.*, 4:15.
10. *Ibid.*, 4:14.
11. *The Ode of Golden Needles*, quoted in Yang Jizhou, *Compendium of Acupuncture and Moxibustion*, p. 56.
12. *Ibid*, p. 56.
13. *Suwen*, 5:48.
14. *Ibid.*, 5:47.
15. *Ibid.*, 5:47.
16. Zhang Zhongjing (*c.* 156–219 AD), *Discussion of Cold-Induced Diseases* (*Shanghan Lun* 伤寒论) (*c.* 200–210 AD). Shanghai: Shanghai People's Press, 1976), p. 27.
17. *Lingshu*, 51:100.
18. Yang Jizhou, *Compendium of Acupuncture and Moxibustion*, p. 122.
19. *Suwen*, 27:170.

> Huang Di asked, 'How do we supplement deficient conditions with acupuncture?' Qi Bo answered, 'When using needling to supplement, first find the acupoint and rub the skin there. Press up and down with your finger to disperse the *qi* in the meridian. Massage the acupoint to stir up its energy. Then ask the patient to focus the attention. Insert the needle when the patient exhales.'

20. Yang Jizhou, *Compendium of Acupuncture and Moxibustion*, pp. 102–122.
21. Dou Hanqing, *Lyrics of Standard Profundities*, quoted in Yang Jizhou, *Compendium of Acupuncture and Moxibustion*, p. 42.
22. *Lingshu*, 1:2.

23. *Lingshu*, 73:131–133.

> Huang Di's minister Lei Gong asked: 'How should occupations be appointed according to ability?' Huang Di answered: 'Appoint those who have sharp eyes to observe the five colors [i.e. visual examination]. Appoint those who have good ears to listen to voices [i.e. aural examination]. Appoint those who have a glib tongue to teach basic theories. Appoint those who are soft-spoken, contained, skillful, and attentive to practice acupuncture and moxibustion, to regulate the flow of *qi* and blood, to identify yin and yang, or to grasp several therapies concurrently. Appoint those who have relaxed joints, pliable muscles and tendons, and an even-temper to practice *daoyin* [physical exercises] and *xingqi* [breathing exercises]. Appoint those who like to slander and look down on others to practice *zhuyou* [incantation], especially for the treatment of *yong* conditions [furuncle]. Appoint those who usually use too much force and damage utensils easily to practice massage for treatment of masses and *bi* syndrome. If only people are appointed according to their ability and specialty, various therapeutic methods can be popularized and those who instruct them will be well-known.'

24. Dou Hanqing, *Lyrics of Standard Profundities*, quoted in Yang Jizhou, *Compendium of Acupuncture and Moxibustion*, p. 43.
25. *Ode of Golden Needles*, quoted in Yang Jizhou, *Compendium of Acupuncture and Moxibustion*, p. 56.
26. *Suwen*, 27:170.
27. Zhu Lian, *New Acupuncture and Moxibustion*, p. 17.
28. *Suwen*, 25:162–163.
29. Tang De'an *et al.*, *Experimental Acupuncture and Moxibustion*, pp. 79–80.
30. Many Westerners think of acupuncture as being synonymous with acupuncture anesthesia. In reality, the use of acupuncture as an anesthetic is a relatively new development. In 1958, drawing inspiration from acupuncture's pain-relieving applications, Chinese practitioners started to use acupuncture to control postoperative pain, and later experimented with it as an anesthetic for simple operations such as tonsillitis and oral surgery. This technique was found to be effective and its applications expanded quickly. In China acupuncture is now used for anesthesia during a wide variety of minor and major operations, as well as prior to and following surgery.
31. See Ted J. Kaptchuk, *Chinese Medicine – The Web that has no Weaver*, pp. 111–112, for an overview of studies on pain relief using acupuncture.
32. *Lingshu*, 5:18.
33. *Lingshu*, 4:14.

> Small pulses of the five *zang* organs indicate deficiency of the body's yin and yang *qi*. Treat this condition with tonifying sweet herbs, not with needles.

Appendix 1

The *Ancient Medical Relics of Mawangdui*

Introduction

In late 1973, a number of ancient documents concerning early Chinese history, philosophy, geography, military affairs, astronomy, divination and medicine were excavated from Grave No. 3 at Mawangdui, located on the outskirts of Changsha, Hunan Province. These extremely valuable archeological finds included fourteen medical documents, known collectively as the *Ancient Medical Relics of Mawangdui*. Ten of these documents were hand-copied on silk, and four were written on bamboo slips. No authors are mentioned. Most of the documents were untitled, and were subsequently named according to their subjects or keywords.

The *Ancient Medical Relics of Mawangdui* were probably lost during the Eastern Han Dynasty (25–220 AD), since no references to them have been found after this time. Although the exact age of the documents has not been determined, a wooden tablet found in the grave states that the deceased, the son of Prime Minister Li Chang of the State of Changsha, was buried on February 24, 168 BC, establishing that they were written prior to this date. However, the unsystematic and empirical nature of the contents of the *Relics* has led scholars to believe that they were actually written substantially earlier, probably around the middle of the Warring States Period (475–221 BC)[1]. In any event, the *Ancient Medical Relics of Mawangdui* predate the *Neijing* (*c*. 104–32 BC), making them the oldest medical documents in existence.

Synopses of the fourteen documents of the *Ancient Medical Relics of Mawangdui*

1. Classic of Moxibustion with Eleven Foot-Arm Meridians (Zubi Shiyi Maijiujing 足臂十一脉灸经) *(silk)*
Summary: Distribution and disorders of eleven of the twelve Foot and Arm Regular Meridians, including six Foot Meridians and five of the six Arm Meridians (Arm Jueyin is not included).

Therapeutic method: Moxibustion.

Remarks: The earliest extant medical monograph on meridian theory and moxibustion.

2. Classic of Moxibustion with Eleven Yin-Yang Meridians (Yinyang Shiyi Maijiujing 阴阳十一脉灸经*) (silk)*

Summary: Distribution and disorders of eleven of the twelve Yin and Yang Regular Meridians, including six Yang Meridians and five of the six Yin Meridians (Hand Jueyin is not included).

Three versions of this document have been found, two written on silk and unearthed at Mawangdui, and one inscribed on bamboo slips and excavated at Zhangjiashan, Hubei Province, in 1983.

The *Classic of Moxibustion with Eleven Yin-Yang Meridians* further developed the material found in the *Classic of Moxibustion with Eleven Foot-Arm Meridians*, and served as a primary source for the later *Neijing* (*c.* 104–32 BC). The *Classic of Moxibustion with Eleven Yin-Yang Meridians* differs from the *Neijing* in its naming of the three Hand Yang Meridians, referring to the Hand Taiyang Meridian as the Shoulder Meridian, the Hand Shaoyang Meridian as the Ear Meridian, and the Hand Yangming Meridian as the Tooth Meridian.

Therapeutic method: Moxibustion.

Remarks: An important medical monograph on meridian theory and moxibustion, following the *Classic of Moxibustion with Eleven Foot-Arm Meridians* and preceding the *Neijing*.

3. Methods of Pulse Examination and Bian Stone (Mai Fa 脉法*) (silk)*

Summary: Diagnostic and therapeutic methods. Diagnosis by examining pulse in the area superior to the inner malleolus. Incision of abscess with *bian* stone and four kinds of improper manipulations. Recommends cooling the head and warming the feet to maintain good health, because the head is yang and the feet are yin; yang *qi* is beneficial to the lower but harmful to the upper.

Therapeutic principle: Reinforce deficiency and reduce excess.

Remarks: The earliest extant monograph on pulse diagnosis and *bian* stone therapy.

4. Indications of Death on the Yin-Yang Meridians (Yinyang Mai Sihou 阴阳脉死候*) (silk)*

Summary: Predicts death by inspection of Yin and Yang Meridians.

Therapeutic methods: Recommends exercise to maintain more *qi* in the four limbs than in the five *zang* organs. Good health will result, just as running water is never stale and a swinging door hinge never rusts.

Therapeutic principles: Application of reducing method for excessive pulse and reinforcing method for deficient pulse.

5. Therapeutic Methods for 52 Diseases (Wushi'er Bingfang 五十二病方*) (silk)*

Summary: Fifty-two diseases are discussed (three missing from existing records). The majority are surgical and internal problems; the remainder are pediatric, gynecological and ophthalmic.

Therapeutic methods: A number of methods are given for each condition. Herbal therapy is the primary treatment, with 254 kinds of herbs and 280 prescriptions extant. Various alternative methods are also discussed, including: moxibustion; application of hot compress, dry heat, and steam; hot water baths; horn cupping; massage; *bian* stone therapy; surgery; and *zhuyou* (incantation). Discusses many specific shamanistic techniques.

Remarks: The earliest extant monograph on therapeutic methods, with an emphasis on herbal prescriptions.

6. Prescriptions for Maintaining Health (Yang Sheng Fang 养生方*) (silk)*
Summary: Prescriptions for sexual problems, including impotence (especially in the elderly), swelling of the external genitals, and insufficient semen. Prescriptions for increasing sexuality ability, correcting general deficiency and keeping fit. Includes various sexual techniques; diagram of external female genitals.
    Remarks: The earliest extant monograph on prescriptions for maintaining sexual health.

7. Miscellaneous Prescriptions (Zaliao Fang 杂疗方*) (silk)*
Summary: Prescriptions for deficiency of *qi*, yin and yang. Prescriptions for bee and snake bites.

8. Book of Pregnancy and Delivery (Taichan Shu 胎产书*) (silk)*
Summary: Special care during pregnancy – diet, emotions and environment. Methods to safeguard embryo and fetus, by month. Prescriptions for infertility.
    Remarks: The earliest extant monograph on pregnancy and safeguarding the fetus.

9. Methods for Eliminating Food and Eating Qi (Quegu Shiqi Fang 却谷食气方*) (silk)*
Summary: Therapeutic principle – regulation of diet to maintain health. Grains are eliminated, and a diet of herbs, fruits, vegetables, minerals and water adhered to.
    Therapeutic methods: Consumption of *qi* to maintain health. *Qi* is the energy that animates the body and supports the functioning of its tissues and organs. Consuming *qi* is a type of *qigong* that consists of completely exhaling turbid *qi* and inhaling as much clear *qi* as possible.
    Remarks: This is the earliest extant monograph to present specific methods for regulating diet and consuming *qi*.

10. Maps of Daoyin (Daoyin Tu 导引图*) (silk)*
Summary: *Daoyin* is a type of physical exercise that combines breathing exercises and self-massage. Forty-four color pictures illustrate various physical exercises, many of which imitate movements of animals.
    Remarks: Contains the earliest extant illustrations of *daoyin* exercises.

11. Ten Questions (Shi Wen 十问*) (bamboo slips)*
Summary: Ten dialogues between Emperors and their subjects, concerning sexual techniques, breathing exercises and diet.
    Remarks: One of the earliest extant documents on sexual techniques.

12. Book of Sex (He Yinyang 合阴阳*) (bamboo slips)*
Summary: Preparation for sexual activity, signs of sexual arousal, and various sexual techniques.
    Remarks: One of the earliest extant monographs on sexual techniques.

13. Miscellaneous Forbidden Methods (Zajin Fang 杂禁方*) (bamboo slips)*
Summary: Various shamanistic methods to promote family harmony, avoid nightmares, stop children's crying.

14. Profound Principle of the Universe (Tianxia Zhidao Tan 天下至道谈*) (bamboo slips)*
Summary: The contents of this book are similar to the *Book of Sex*.
    Remarks: One of the earliest extant monographs on sexual techniques.

References

1. Ma Jixing, *Study and Annotation of Ancient Medical Relics of Mawangdui* (*Mawangdui Guyishu Kaoshi* 马王堆古医书考释). Changsha: Hunan Science and Technology Press, 1992, p. 8.

Appendix 2

The *Classic of Moxibustion with Eleven Foot-Arm Meridians*

Introduction

The *Classic of Moxibustion with Eleven Foot-Arm Meridians* is one of the fourteen ancient documents comprising the *Ancient Medical Relics of Mawangdui*, excavated in 1973 from a burial site dated February 24, 168 BC, located in Mawangdui, Changsha, Hunan Province. The original document had no title, and was named following its discovery according to its contents. The *Classic of Moxibustion with Eleven Foot-Arm Meridians* consists of two parts, which discuss the distribution and diseases of the six Foot Meridians and five of the six Arm Meridians (Arm Jueyin is not included). This and a second document from Mawangdui are the two oldest known monographs on meridian theory and moxibustion.

Throughout the following text descriptions of the Foot and Arm Meridians, the symbol × is used to indicate that the original Chinese character used here has been lost or is unknown. One '×' represents one Chinese character.

Foot Meridians

1. Foot Taiyang Meridian

The Foot Taiyang Meridian originates at the depression posterior to the outer malleolus. It runs upward along the back of the leg and arrives at the popliteal fossa. A branch splits off from the popliteal fossa, and continues upward to spread to the muscles lateral to the lower back.

The main course ascends from the popliteal fossa to pass through the buttock. It then runs upward lateral to the spinal column and the back of the neck, and arrives at the top of the head. Another branch splits off from the head, descends to the forehead and then turns back to the ear. The main course goes directly forward from the top of the head, to pass through the inner canthus and terminate at the nasal region.

If the meridian is diseased, there will be motor impairment of the little toe, pain at the back of the leg, spasm in the popliteal region, pain of the buttocks, hemorrhoids, lower back pain, pain bilateral to the spine, pain at ×, pain on the back of the neck, headache, cold sensation on the forehead, deafness, pain of the eyes, nasal discharge or obstruction, epistaxis, and frequent epileptic attacks. For all diseases mentioned above, apply moxibustion to the Foot Taiyang Meridian.

2. Foot Shaoyang Meridian

The Foot Shaoyang Meridian originates at the front of the outer malleolus. It ascends between the tibia and fibula, passes through the lateral side of the knee and thigh, and arrives at the hypochondriac region.

A branch diverges from the main course at the hypochondriac region to spread to the scapular region. The main course passes through the axillary region, ascends to the back of the neck and ear, arrives at ×, and ends at the outer canthus.

If the meridian is diseased, there will be motor impairment of the fourth toe, pain on the external side of the leg, coldness of the leg; pain on the external side of the knee, thigh and hip; pain in the hypochondriac region, headache, pain on the back of the neck, lumps in the axillary region, pain in the supraclavicular fossa, swelling and pain on the lateral side of the neck, deafness, pain on the occipital region, pain anterior to the ear, pain of the outer canthus, and swelling in the hypochondriac region. For all diseases mentioned above, apply moxibustion to the Foot Shaoyang Meridian.

3. Foot Yangming Meridian

The Foot Yangming Meridian runs upward within the leg, passes through the knee joint, and ascends along the front of the thigh. It then continues upward along the lateral side of the lower abdomen, runs along the medial side of the breast, passes through the throat, goes around the mouth, and ends at the nasal region.

If the meridian is diseased, there will be motor impairment of the middle toe, leg pain, swelling of the knee joint, distension in the abdomen, pain on the medial side of the breast, swelling on the lateral side of ×, pain in the zygomatic region, nasal discharge or obstruction, epistaxis, frequent epileptic attacks, fever and profuse sweating, itching at the external genital region, and facial coldness. For all diseases mentioned above, apply moxibustion to the Foot Yangming Meridian.

4. Foot Shaoyin Meridian

The Foot Shaoyin Meridian originates at the depression posterior to the inner malleolus. It ascends along the medial side of the leg, enters the popliteal fossa, and continues along the medial side of the thigh. The meridian continues upward to enter the abdominal cavity, ascends along the inside of the spine, connects with the liver, and spreads to the hypochondriac region. It finally ascends to connect with the root of the tongue.

If the meridian is diseased, there will be a sensation of heat in the feet, pain at the medial side of the leg and thigh, pain in the inguinal region, pain inside the spinal column, pain of the liver, heartache, restlessness, throat × × ×, dry tongue with crackles on its surface, × jaundice, shortness of breath, × ×, asthma with throat rattle, muteness, drowsiness, and cough. For all diseases mentioned above, apply moxibustion to the Foot Shaoyin Meridian.

5. Foot Taiyin Meridian

The Foot Taiyin Meridian originates at the medial side of the big toe. It runs upward along the upper side of the inner malleolus, and ascends along the medial side of the leg, knee and thigh.

If the meridian is diseased, there will be motor impairment of the big toe, pain in the medial side of the leg and thigh, abdominal pain and distension, ×, poor appetite, frequent belching, restlessness and palpitation. For all diseases mentioned above, apply moxibustion to the Foot Taiyin Meridian.

6. Foot Jueyin Meridian

The Foot Jueyin Meridian passes through the space between the great and second toes on the dorsum of the foot. It then ascends along the medial side of the leg. At 8 *cun* above the inner malleolus, the meridian crosses the Foot Taiyin Meridian. It continues upward along the medial side of the thigh and arrives at the external genital region.

If the meridian is diseased, there will be itching in the external genital region, frequent urination, thirst and preference for drinks, swelling on the dorsum of foot, and *bi* syndrome [i.e. pain of the joints]. For all diseases mentioned above, apply moxibustion to the Foot Jueyin Meridian.

Arm Meridians

1. Arm Taiyin Meridian

The Arm Taiyin Meridian runs upward along the upper border of the tendon [i.e. the radial flexor muscle of the wrist], ascends to the medial side of the upper arm, emerges on the medial side of the axillary fossa, and enters the thoracic cavity to connect with the heart.

If the meridian is diseased, there will be heartache, restlessness and eructation. For all diseases mentioned above, apply moxibustion to the Arm Taiyin Meridian.

2. Arm Shaoyin Meridian

The Arm Shaoyin Meridian runs upward along the lower border of the tendon [i.e. the ulnar flexor muscle of the wrist]. It continues upward along the posterior border of the medial side of the upper arm, emerges in the axillary region, and arrives at the hypochondriac region.

If the meridian is diseased, there will be pain in the hypochondriac region. For this disease, apply moxibustion to the Arm Shaoyin Meridian.

3. Arm Taiyang Meridian

The Arm Taiyang Meridian originates at the little finger. It runs upward on the external side of the forearm along the lower border of the lower bone [i.e. the ulna] and the posterior border of the external side of the upper arm. It then spreads to the back of the shoulder, ascends to the lateral side of the neck, × × ×, and finally arrives at the outer canthus.

If the meridian is diseased, there will be pain on the external side of the upper limb. For this disease, apply moxibustion to the Hand Taiyang Meridian.

4. Arm Shaoyang Meridian

The Arm Shaoyang Meridian originates at the middle finger. It runs upward on the external side of the forearm along the lower border of the upper bone [i.e. the radius], and finally arrives at the ear.

If the meridian is diseased, there will be deafness and cheek pain. For diseases mentioned above, apply moxibustion to the Hand Shaoyang Meridian.

5. Arm Yangming Meridian

The Arm Yangming Meridian originates from the space between the index and middle fingers. It ascends on the external side of the forearm along the upper border [i.e. the radial side] of the radius and the external side of the upper arm. It continues upward to × and arrives at the mouth.

If the meridian is diseased, there will be toothache, × ×, and × ×. For all diseases mentioned above, apply moxibustion to the Arm Yangming Meridian.

In conclusion, there are six Foot Meridians and five Hand Meridians.

Appendix 3

The *Classic of Moxibustion with Eleven Yin-Yang Meridians*

Introduction

The *Classic of Moxibustion with Eleven Yin-Yang Meridians* is the second of two monographs on meridian theory and moxibustion included in the fourteen *Ancient Medical Relics of Mawangdui*. These two documents are the oldest known monographs on meridian theory and moxibustion. The original document had no title, and was named following its discovery according to its contents. The *Classic of Moxibustion with Eleven Yin-Yang Meridians* consists of two parts, which discuss the six Yang meridians and five of the six Yin meridians (Hand Jueyin is not included). Three versions of this document have been found, two written on silk and unearthed at Mawangdui, and one written on bamboo slips and excavated at Zhangjiashan, Hubei Province in 1983.

The *Classic of Moxibustion with Eleven Yin-Yang Meridians* differs from the *Classic of Moxibustion with Eleven Foot-Arm Meridians* and the *Neijing* in its naming of the three Hand Yang Meridians. It refers to the Hand Taiyang Meridian as the Shoulder Meridian, the Hand Shaoyang Meridian as the Ear Meridian, and the Hand Yangming as the Tooth Meridian. There is a close relationship among the distribution and indications of these meridians and the names given to them by the *Classic of Moxibustion with Eleven Yin-Yang Meridians*. For instance, the Shoulder Meridian distributes on the shoulder, and is used for problems such as frozen shoulder. The acupoints of the three Hand Yang Meridians are very important for treating diseases of the shoulder, ear and teeth respectively.

Throughout the following text descriptions of the Yang and Yin Meridians, the symbol × is used to indicate that the original Chinese character used here has been lost or is unknown. One '×' represents one Chinese character.

Yang Meridians

1. Foot Taiyang Meridian
The Foot Taiyang Meridian originates from the depression between the outer malleolus and the heel. It runs upward along the back of the lower limb, passes through the popliteal fossa and buttock, and emerges above the depression on the buttock [i.e. the area of the great trochanter]. It continues upward along the lateral side of the spine and the back of the neck, and arrives at the top of the head. It then goes forward to the forehead, descends to the lateral side of the bridge of the nose, and connects with the inner canthus.

If the meridian is diseased, there will be severe headache; pain, distension and a dropping feeling in the eyeballs; rigidity and a pulling feeling in the neck; pain of the spine; splitting pain in the lumbar region; motor impairment of the hip joint; rigidity and freezing up of the popliteal region; and splitting pain on the back of the leg. All these diseases are due to *qi* reversal at the ankle region, and are indications of the Foot Taiyang Meridian.

Dysfunction of the meridian may lead to headache, deafness, pain on the back of the neck, stiff neck, malaria, backache, lumbar pain, pain of the buttocks, hemorrhoids, pain in the popliteal region, pain on the back of the leg, and motor impairment of the little toe. There are a total of twelve disorders.

2. Foot Shaoyang Meridian

The Foot Shaoyang Meridian originates in front of the outer malleolus. It ascends to the external side of the thigh, passes through the hypochondriac region, and terminates at the region inferior to the eye.

If the meridian is diseased, there will be pain in the precordial and hypochondriac regions, aggravated by turning over in bed; rough, dry, dull skin in severe cases; and strephexopodia. All these diseases are due to yang reversal of the Foot Shaoyang Meridian, and are indications of Foot Shaoyang Meridian.

Dysfunction of the meridian may lead to × × ×, pain in the head and neck, pain in the hypochondriac region, malaria, sweating, joint pain, pain on the external side of the thigh, pain of ×, pain on the front of the thigh, pain on the external side of the knee, chills, and motor impairment of the middle toe. There are a total of twelve disorders. Additionally, there may be fever.

3. Foot Yangming Meridian

The Foot Yangming Meridian runs along the lateral side of the tibia. It goes upward to penetrate the knee joint, and ascends along the lateral side of the muscles on the front of the thigh. The meridian continues upward, passes through the breast and cheek, arrives at the outer canthus, and goes around the forehead.

If the meridian is diseased, there will be chills, frequent stretching, repeated yawning, dark complexion on the forehead, edema, aversion to company and heat at onset, fear at hearing the sound of tapping on wood, palpitations, and desire to stay in a sealed room [i.e. agoraphobia]. In severe cases, the patient may climb up on a table and sing, or even disrobe and engage in unruly acts. All of these conditions are due to *qi* reversal in the leg region, and are also indications of the Foot Yangming Meridian.

Dysfunction of the Foot Yangming Meridian may lead to frontal headache, nasal discharge or obstruction, pain in the area below the lower jaw and neck, pain in the breasts, pain in the precordal and hypochondriac regions, abdominal distension, pain in the intestines, rigidity of the knee joint, and numbness and pain on the dorsum of the foot. There are a total of ten disorders.

4. Shoulder Meridian

The Shoulder Meridian originates behind the ear. It descends to the shoulder, runs along the external side of the upper arm and forearm, passes through the wrist, and arrives at the dorsum of the hand.

If the Shoulder Meridian is diseased, there will be sore throat, pain and swelling below the lower jaw and resulting difficulty in turning the head, severe dropping pain in the shoulder, and pain in the upper arm as if being broken. All these diseases are indications of the Shoulder Meridian.

Dysfunction of the meridian may lead to pain below the lower jaw, swelling and pain of the throat, pain of the upper limb, and pain on the external side of the elbow. There are a total of four conditions.

5. Ear Meridian
The Ear Meridian starts from the dorsum of the hand. It runs upward along the external side of the forearm between the two bones [i.e. the radius and ulna] and along the approximate lower border of the upper bone [i.e. the radius]. The meridian continues upward to pass through the center of the elbow, and finally enters the ear.

If the meridian is diseased, there will be deafness, thunderous ringing in the ears, and swelling of the throat. These problems are indications of the Ear Meridian.

Dysfunction of the Ear Meridian may lead to pain at the outer canthus, cheek pain and deafness. There are a total of three disorders.

6. Tooth Meridian
The Tooth Meridian originates at the space between the index finger and thumb. It runs upward along the upper border of the forearm, passes through the elbow, ascends along the external side of the upper arm, penetrates the cheek, enters the teeth, and terminates at the side of the nose.

If the meridian is diseased, there will be toothache and swelling on the zygomatic region. These problems are indications of the Tooth Meridian.

Dysfunction of the meridian may lead to toothache, swelling on the zygomatic region, yellow eyes, dry mouth and pain of the upper arm. There are a total of five disorders. Additionally, there may be × ×× ×.

Yin Meridians

1. Foot Taiyin Meridian
The Foot Taiyin Meridian is also known as the Stomach Meridian. It originates at the stomach, descends along the posterior border of the medial side of the thigh and the anterior border of the medial side of the leg, and arrives at the region anterior to the inner malleolus.

If the meridian is diseased, there will be attack on the heart by uprising *qi* [marked by palpitation and fright], abdominal distension, frequent eructation, and vomiting induced by intake of food. All these symptoms will be immediately alleviated after defecation or breaking wind. They are indications of the Foot Taiyin Meridian.

Dysfunction of the Foot Taiyin Meridian may lead to × ×, restlessness, pain in the heart region, abdominal distension, poor appetite, discomfort when lying down [due to abdominal distension], yawning, loose stool or diarrhea, edema and retention of urine. There are a total of ten disorders.

2. Foot Jueyin Meridian
The Foot Jueyin Meridian originates at the hairy region on the top of the big toe. It runs upward along the top of the foot, and ascends to the medial side of the leg from the area anterior to the inner malleolus. At 5 *cun* above the inner malleolus, the meridian crosses the Foot Taiyin Meridian and then passes behind it. It continues upward along the medial side of the muscles in front of the thigh, enters the lower abdomen, and finally ends at the inner canthus.

If the meridian is diseased, there will be swelling and pain of the testes in the male, lower abdominal pain and distension in the female, lumbar pain aggravated by lying on the back, and possibly dry throat and a dark facial complexion in severe cases. These are indications of the Foot Jueyin Meridian.

Dysfunction of the Foot Jueyin Meridian may lead to a sensation of heat inside the body, retention of urine, swelling and pain of the testes in the case of the male, inguinal hernia, and × ×. There are a total of five disorders.

3. Foot Shaoyin Meridian
The Foot Shaoyin Meridian originates behind the inner malleolus. It ascends along the medial side of the leg and exits from the center of the popliteal fossa. The meridian continues upward to enter the abdominal cavity, and proceeds along the inside of the spine. It connects with the kidney within the abdominal cavity, and then ascends to end at the lateral side of the root of the tongue.

If the meridian is diseased, there will be depression, restlessness, blurred vision when suddenly standing up from a sitting position, palpitation and dropping sensation of the heart, frequent hunger, *qi* deficiency, fear with the feeling of being pursued, poor appetite, a dull sooty facial complexion, and coughing of blood. These diseases are due to *qi* reversal of the bones, and are indications of the Foot Shaoyin Meridian.

Dysfunction of the meridian may lead to a sensation of heat in the mouth, a dry tongue with a cracked surface, dry throat, shortness of breath, difficulty in swallowing, sore throat, jaundice, drowsiness, cough and hoarseness. There are a total of ten disorders.

When applying moxibustion to the Foot Shaoyin Meridian, the patient should be directed to eat raw meat, keep the belt loose and the hair unbound, and to use a stout cane and sturdy shoes. The diseases will be cured after several treatments with moxibustion.

4. Arm Taiyin Meridian
The Arm Taiyin Meridian originates at the palm of the hand. It ascends between the two bones [i.e. radius and ulna] on the medial side of the forearm, approximately between the ulnar side of the radius and the tendon [i.e. the radial flexor muscle of the wrist]. It then continues upward along the medial side of the upper arm, and finally enters the cavity to the heart.

If the meridian is diseased, there will be rapid heartbeat and pain in the heart, pain in the supraclavicular fossa, and even extreme chills in severe cases. All these diseases are due to *qi* reversal at the forearm region, and are indications of the Arm Taiyin Meridian.

Dysfunction of the Arm Taiyin Meridian will lead to pain in the chest, epigastric pain, pain in the heart, pain in the hands and feet, and lumps in the abdomen. There are a total of five disorders.

5. Arm Shaoyin Meridian
The Arm Shaoyin Meridian originates between the two bones [i.e. ulna and radius] on the medial side of the forearm. It ascends between the radial side of the ulna and the tendon [i.e. the ulnar flexor muscle of the wrist], continues upward along the medial side of the upper arm, and finally enters the heart.

If the meridian is diseased, there will be heartache, dry throat, thirst, and desire for liquids. All these diseases are due to *qi* reversal at the forearm, and are indications of the Arm Shaoyin Meridian.

Dysfunction of the Arm Shaoyin Meridian will lead to pain in the hypochondriac region. There is only one condition.

In conclusion, there are a total of twenty-two meridians – twelve bilateral Yang Meridians and ten bilateral Yin Meridians – and seventy-seven related diseases.

Appendix 4

Chapter 10 of the *Lingshu*: 'Meridians'

Introduction

Lingshu – the Spiritual Pivot (Lingshujing), also known as *The Classic of Acupuncture (Zhenjing* 针经), comprises the first, and older, half of the *Neijing – The Yellow Emperor's Inner Classic of Medicine (Huang Di Neijing)* (*c.* 104–32 BC). Chapter 10 of the *Lingshu*, 'Meridians (*Jingmai*)', is one of the most important sections of the *Neijing*, the seminal work of traditional Chinese medicine. Up until the discovery of the *Ancient Medical Relics of Mawangdui* (*c.* prior to 168 BC), 'Meridians' provided the earliest known exposition of the distribution and indications of the twelve Regular Meridians, and was used as the sole reference on meridian theory in all books on acupuncture.

A comparison of content indicates that the authors of the *Neijing* used the *Classic of Moxibustion with Eleven Foot-Arm Meridians* and the *Classic of Moxibustion with Eleven Yin-Yang Meridians* from the *Ancient Medical Relics of Mawangdui*, now recognized as the oldest extant writings on the meridians, as primary references. Of course, the *Neijing* did not simply reproduce these earlier documents, but rather refined and developed them, and introduced new therapeutic methods. In addition to the eleven Regular Meridians discussed in the two older texts, 'Meridians' introduced the Pericardium Meridian of Hand Jueyin, bringing the number of Regular Meridians to the twelve we know today. Furthermore, the *Neijing* expanded the system of twelve Regular Meridians internally to include the twelve corresponding *zangfu* organs, and externally to form an interconnected circular network.

The most important difference between the two earlier texts on the meridians and Chapter 10 of the *Lingshu*, however, lies in their respective therapeutic methods. The former is limited to moxibustion, while 'Meridians' mentions needling therapy, or acupuncture, for the first time in recorded history. 'Meridians' took meridian theory one step further, ushering in the rapid development of acupuncture that was shortly to follow, when it stated in its very first sentence: 'Meridian theory is the basis of all principles of acupuncture'.

Excerpts of text

1. Lung Meridian of Hand Taiyin
The Lung Meridian of Hand Taiyin originates within the Middle Jiao. It runs downward to connect with the large intestine. Winding back, it goes upward alongside the upper

orifice of the stomach, penetrates the diaphragm, and enters the thoracic cavity to connect with the lungs, its pertaining *zang* organ. It then runs transversely to emerge from the axillary region at *feixi*, the tissues which connect the lungs with the other *zangfu* organs. The meridian then runs downward along the medial side of the upper arm, passing in front of the Hand Shaoyin and Hand Jueyin Meridians. After passing through the middle of the elbow, the meridian continues downward along the medial side of the forearm along the lower border of the radius [i.e. the ulnar side of the radius], and thence through *cunkou* [i.e. the radial artery area of the wrist where the pulse is taken]. It then runs along the radial edge of the thenar eminence, and ends at the radial side of the tip of the thumb.

A branch of the Lung Meridian diverges from the main course just above the wrist. The branch runs along the radial side of the index finger and ends at the radial side of the tip of the index finger.

If the meridian is diseased, there will be a feeling of distension in the chest, asthma with throat rattle, cough, pain in the supraclavicular fossa, and even extreme chills in severe cases. These diseases are due to *qi* reversal in the forearm region.

The Lung Meridian is indicated for treatment of disorders due to lung dysfunction, including cough, difficulty in inhaling, asthma with throat rattle, restlessness, feeling of fullness in the chest, pain and coldness on the anterior side of the upper limb, and sensation of heat in the palm.

In cases of excessive evil *qi*, there will be pain in the shoulder and arm, sweating when attacked by wind-cold, and frequent but scanty urination. In cases of deficient right *qi*, there will be pain and sensation of cold in the shoulder and upper back, shortness of breath, and color change of the urine.

2. Large Intestine Meridian of Hand Yangming

The Large Intestine Meridian of Hand Yangming starts at the tip of the index finger, runs upward along the radial side of the index finger, and passes through the interspace of the first and second metacarpal bones. It then dips into the depression between two tendons of the thumb [i.e. the long and short extensor muscles of the thumb]. The meridian continues upward along the anterior border of the external side of the upper limb to the top of the shoulder. Passing along the anterior border of the acromion, it arrives at the seventh cervical vertebra [i.e. DU14-Dazhui], the meeting point of all Hand and Foot Yang Meridians. The meridian then winds back and enters the body cavity through the supraclavicular fossa. Within the cavity, it connects with the lungs, passes through the diaphragm, and finally connects with the large intestine, its pertaining *fu* organ.

A branch of the Large Intestine Meridian diverges from the main course at the supraclavicular fossa. The branch ascends externally along the lateral side of the neck, penetrates the lower jaw, and enters the lower teeth. The bilateral sides of the meridian then emerge to curve around the mouth and cross at the philtrum. From there, the left side of the meridian runs to the right and the right to the left, ending at the areas lateral to the wings of the nose.

If the meridian is diseased, there will be toothache and swelling of the neck.

The Large Intestine Meridian is indicated for treatment of disorders due to disturbance of the *jin* or dilute bodily fluids, including yellow eyes, dry mouth, nasal discharge or obstruction, epistaxis, swelling and pain of the throat, pain on the anterior external side of the shoulder and upper arm, and motor impairment of the index finger.

In cases of excessive evil *qi*, there will be heat and swelling along the external pathway of the meridian. In cases of deficient right *qi*, there will be a persistent feeling of cold and shivering.

3. Stomach Meridian of Foot Yangming

The Stomach Meridian of Foot Yangming begins at the lateral side of the wing of the nose. It then ascends to the bridge of the nose and meets the Urinary Bladder Meridian at the inner canthus. Descending from there, the meridian runs lateral to the nose and enters the upper teeth. It then curves around the lips, meeting the Ren Meridian at the mentolabial groove. Winding back from the groove, it goes along the lower side of the lower jawbone and passes through the angle of the mandible. The meridian then ascends to run in front of the ear, passing through *Kezhuren* (i.e. GB2–Shangguan), and terminates at the outer corner of the forehead.

A branch of the Stomach Meridian diverges from the main course at the lower jaw. The branch descends along the lateral side of the throat, passes through *Renying* (i.e. the common carotid artery), and enters the thoracic cavity through the supraclavicular fossa. The branch continues downward through the thoracic cavity, and passes through the diaphragm to the abdomen, where it connects with the stomach, its pertaining *fu* organ, and the spleen.

From the point where the branch diverges at the lower jaw, the main course of the Stomach Meridian runs directly downward from the supraclavicular fossa, remaining on the surface of the body. It passes through the breast and lateral side of the umbilicus and arrives at the inguinal region.

Internally, a branch of the Stomach Meridian diverges from the main course at the lower outlet of the stomach [i.e. pylorus], descends through the abdomen, and emerges from the inguinal region where it rejoins the main course. From this point, the main course runs downward on the surface through the hip joint to the knee joint. It continues downward along the external side of the tibia, passes through the dorsum of the foot, and arrives at the space medial to the middle toe.

An additional branch of the Stomach Meridian diverges from the main course 3 *cun* below the knee joint. It descends to the space lateral to the middle toe.

The final branch of the Stomach Meridian diverges from the main course on the top of the foot. It runs to the big toe and terminates at its tip.

If the meridian is diseased, there will be chills, frequent stretching, repeated yawning, dark complexion on the forehead, aversion to company and fire during the early stages, fear at hearing the sound of tapping wood, palpitation, and desire to stay in a sealed room [i.e. agoraphobia]. In severe cases, the patient may get up on a table and sing, or even disrobe and engage in unruly behavior. There will also be hiccuping and abdominal distension. All these diseases are due to *qi* reversal in the leg region.

The Stomach Meridian is indicated for treatment of disorders due to disturbances of the blood, including mania, malaria, febrile diseases, sweating, nasal discharge or obstruction, epistaxis, deviation of the mouth, ulcers of the lips, swelling of the neck, swelling and pain of the throat, abdominal distension, edema, and swelling and pain of the knee joint; as well as pain along the external pathway of the meridian, including the chest, breast, inguinal region, front of the thigh, external side of the leg, and dorsum of the foot. There will also be motor impairment of the middle toe.

In cases of excessive evil *qi*, there will be a sensation of heat in the front of the body; if there is excessive evil *qi* in the stomach, there will be swift digestion quickly followed by hunger and yellow urine. In cases of deficient right *qi*, there will be low tolerance to cold along the front of the body; if there is cold in the stomach, there will be epigastric distension.

4. Spleen Meridian of Foot Taiyin

The Spleen Meridian of Foot Taiyin starts at the medial side of the tip of the big toe. It runs along the medial side of the toe at the junction of the red and white skin (i.e. the junction of the top and bottom of the foot). After passing through the first metatarsal bone, the meridian ascends in front of the medial malleolus to the medial side of the leg. It continues upward along the posterior edge of the tibia, and passes in front of the Foot Jueyin Meridian. Ascending along the anterior border of the medial side of the knee and thigh, it enters the abdominal cavity to connect with the spleen, its pertaining *zang* organ, and the stomach. The meridian then passes through the diaphragm, and runs alongside the esophagus and throat. It finally connects with the root of the tongue, and spreads over its lower surface.

A branch of the Spleen Meridian diverges from the main course at the stomach, passes upward through the diaphragm, and enters the heart.

If the meridian is diseased, there will be rigidity at the root of the tongue, vomiting induced by intake of food, epigastric pain, abdominal distension, and frequent belching. All these symptoms will be immediately alleviated after defecation or breaking wind. There will also be heaviness of the whole body.

The Spleen Meridian is indicated for treatment of disorders due to spleen dysfunction, including pain at the root of the tongue, poor appetite, restlessness, acute pain in the epigastric region, loose stool, lumps in the abdomen, diarrhea, edema, retention of urine, jaundice, difficulty in lying down [due to abdominal distention], swelling and coldness on the front of the knee and thigh after prolonged standing, and motor impairment of the big toe.

5. Heart Meridian of Hand Shaoyin

The Heart Meridian of Hand Shaoyin originates at the heart. It goes upward to connect with *xinxi*, the tissues which connect the heart with the other organs. It then turns downward, and passes through the diaphragm to connect with the small intestine.

A branch of the Heart Meridian diverges from the main course at *xinxi*, the connecting tissues of the heart, ascends alongside the throat, and goes directly upward to connect with *muxi*, the tissues which connect the eyes with the brain.

The main course of the meridian ascends from *xinxi*, the connecting tissues of the heart, to connect with the lungs. It then emerges at the axillary fossa. From there, it descends along the posterior border of the medial side of the upper arm, behind the Hand Taiyin and Hand Jueyin Meridians. Running along the posterior border of the medial side of the elbow and forearm, it arrives at the pisiform region. It then goes along the medial side of the palm and the radial border of the little finger, and terminates at the radial side of the tip of the little finger.

If the meridian is diseased, there will be dry throat, pain in the heart region, thirst, and desire for liquids. These diseases are due to *qi* reversal at the forearm region.

The Heart Meridian is indicated for treatment of problems due to heart dysfunction, including yellow eyes, pain in the hypochondriac region, pain and coldness on the posterior border of the medial side of the forearm and upper arm, and sensation of heat in the palms.

6. Small Intestine Meridian of Hand Taiyang

The Small Intestine Meridian of Hand Taiyang originates at the ulnar side of the tip of the little finger. It then ascends along the ulnar side of the dorsum of the hand, runs upward along the posterior border of the external side of the forearm, and passes through the interspace between the two bones at the elbow region [i.e. the olecranon of the ulna and the medial epicondyle of the humerus]. The meridian continues upward along the posterior border of the external side of the upper arm to the shoulder joint, circles around the scapular region, and meets the Du Meridian at the seventh cervical vertebra [i.e.

DU14-Dazhui]. From there, it turns forward and enters the thoracic cavity through the supraclavicular fossa. After connecting with the heart within the thoracic cavity, the meridian continues downward alongside the esophagus, penetrates the diaphragm, reaches the stomach, and finally connects with the small intestine, its pertaining *fu* organ.

A branch of the Small Intestine Meridian diverges from the main course at the supraclavicular fossa. The branch ascends along the lateral side of the neck, passes through the cheek, connects with the outer canthus, and finally turns back to enter the ear.

Another branch diverges from the main course at the cheek. It runs upward to the infraorbital region and the nose, and terminates at the inner canthus of the eye.

If the meridian is diseased, there will be sore throat, pain and swelling below the lower jaw and resulting difficulty in turning the head, severe dropping pain in the shoulder, and splitting pain in the upper arm.

The Small Intestine Meridian is indicated for treatment of disturbances of the *ye* or sticky bodily fluids, including deafness, yellow eyes, swelling of the cheek, pain of the neck, pain below the lower jaw, shoulder pain, and pain along the posterior border of the external side of the upper limb.

7. Urinary Bladder Meridian of Foot Taiyang

The Urinary Bladder Meridian of Foot Taiyang starts at the inner canthus. It ascends to the forehead, and meets the Du Meridian on the top of the head [i.e. DU20-Baihui].

A short branch of the Urinary Bladder Meridian diverges from the main course at the top of the vertex and descends to the uppermost junction of the auricle and skull.

From the top of the vertex, the main course of the meridian enters the skull to connect with the brain. It then emerges and descends to the back of the neck. The meridian continues downward along the medial border of the scapular region and parallel to the spine. At the lumbar region, it enters the abdominal cavity to connect with the urinary bladder, its pertaining *fu* organ, and the kidney.

A branch of the Urinary Bladder Meridian diverges from the main course at the lumbar region, goes directly downward alongside the spine, passes through the buttock, and enters the popliteal fossa.

Another branch diverges from the main course at the back of the neck. It runs downward along the medial side of the shoulder and passes through the scapula. The branch then continues downward parallel to the spine, and passes through the buttock. Descending along the posterior border of the back of the thigh, this branch joins the preceding branch at the popliteal fossa. From there, the joined branches go downward along the back of the leg, pass through the posterior area of the external malleolus, and run along the lateral side of the foot to reach the lateral side of the tip of the little toe.

If the meridian is diseased, there will be severe headache, dropping pain and distension of the eyeballs, rigidity and pulling sensation in the neck, pain of the spine, severe pain in the lumbar region, motor impairment of the hip joint, immobilizing pain in the popliteal region, and splitting pain on the back of the leg. All these diseases are due to *qi* reversal at the ankle region.

The Urinary Bladder Meridian is indicated for treatment of disorders due to tendon disturbance, including hemorrhoids, malaria, mania, epilepsy, pain on the fontanel and the back of the neck, yellow eyes, lacrimation, nasal discharge or obstruction, and epistaxis; as well as pain along the pathway of the meridian, including the back of the neck, back, lumbar region, buttocks, popliteal fossa, back of the leg, and foot. There will also be motor impairment of the little toe.

8. Kidney Meridian of Foot Shaoyin

The Kidney Meridian of Foot Shaoyin originates on the inferior side of the little toe. It runs across the sole of the foot, emerges from the lower aspect of the tuberosity of the navicular bone, and proceeds to the back of the inner malleolus. From there the meridian enters the heel, where it turns to ascend along the medial side of the leg. Emerging from the medial side of the popliteal fossa, the meridian continues upward to pass through the spine and connect with the kidney, its pertaining *zang* organ, and the urinary bladder.

Within the abdominal cavity, the main course of the meridian ascends from the kidney, passes through the liver and diaphragm, and then enters the lung. It proceeds upward along the throat, and finally ends at the lateral side of the root of the tongue.

A branch of the Kidney Meridian diverges from the main course at the lung area. It connects with the heart, and then distributes to the inside of the chest.

If the meridian is diseased, there will be hunger but no desire for food, a dull sooty facial complexion, coughing of blood, asthma with throat rattle, blurred vision when standing suddenly, heart palpitation with a sensation of dropping or hunger, *qi* deficiency, and fear with the feeling of being pursued. All these diseases are due to *qi* reversal of the bones.

The Kidney Meridian is indicated for treatment of disorders due to kidney dysfunction, including sensation of heat in the mouth, dry tongue, swelling of the throat, shortness of breath, dryness and pain of the throat, restlessness, pain in the heart region, jaundice, diarrhea, pain inside the spinal column, pain along the posterior border of the medial side of the thigh, *wei* syndrome or muscular atrophy, cold limbs, drowsiness, and pain and sensation of heat in the soles of the feet. When applying moxibustion to the Foot Shaoyin Meridian, the patient should be directed to eat raw meat, keep the belt loose and the hair unbound, and to use a stout cane and sturdy shoes.

9. Pericardium Meridian of Hand Jueyin

The Pericardium Meridian of Hand Jueyin originates at the center of the chest. It connects with the pericardium, its pertaining *zang* organ, and then descends through the diaphragm to link consecutively with each of the three San Jiao.

A branch of the Pericardium Meridian diverges from the main course at the chest and emerges in the hypochondriac region. It ascends to the area below the axilla, then descends along the middle of the medial side of the upper arm, passing between the Hand Taiyin and Hand Shaoyin Meridians. After passing through the center of the elbow, the branch continues downward on the middle of the forearm between the two tendons [i.e. the tendons of the long palmar muscle and the radial flexor muscle of wrist]. It then descends through the center of the palm, runs along the palmar side of the middle finger, and terminates at the tip of the middle finger.

Another branch of the Pericardium Meridian diverges from the main course at the palm, and proceeds to the tip of the ring finger.

If the meridian is diseased, there will be a sensation of heat in the palms, contracture of the forearm and elbow, swelling in the axillary region or even distension in the chest and hypochondriac region, rapid heartbeat, reddened facial complexion, yellow eyes, and incessant laughing.

The Pericardium Meridian is indicated for treatment of diseases due to disturbance of the blood vessels, including restlessness, pain in the heart region, and the sensation of heat in the palms.

10. San Jiao Meridian of Hand Shaoyang

The San Jiao Meridian of Hand Shaoyang starts at the tip of the ring finger. It runs upward between the fourth and fifth metacarpal bones on the back of the hand, and between the ulna and radius on the external side of the forearm. The meridian then passes through the elbow, runs along the middle of the external side of the upper arm, and arrives on the top of the shoulder. From here, it crosses behind the Foot Shaoyang Meridian and enters the thoracic cavity through the supraclavicular fossa, distributes to the Upper Jiao, the top third of its pertaining *fu* organ, and connects with the pericardium. It then penetrates the diaphragm to connect with the Middle and Lower Jiao, the lower two-thirds of its pertaining *fu* organ.

A branch of the San Jiao Meridian diverges from the main course inside the chest cavity. The branch goes upward and emerges through the supraclavicular fossa. It continues upward along the lateral side of the neck and behind the ear to the uppermost junction of the auricle and skull, and then turns forward to the cheek and terminates at the infraorbital region.

Another branch splits off behind the ear and enters the ear. It then emerges from the front of the ear, passes through *kezhuren* (i.e. GB2–Shangguan), meets the cheek, and ends at the outer canthus.

If the meridian is diseased, there will be deafness, thunderous ringing in the ears, and swelling and pain of the throat.

The San Jiao Meridian is indicated for treatment of disorders due to *qi* disturbance, including sweating, pain at the outer canthus, swollen cheek, pain behind the ears, and pain on the back of the shoulder and external side of the upper arm, elbow, and forearm. There will also be motor impairment of the index finger.

11. Gallbladder Meridian of Foot Shaoyang
The Gallbladder Meridian of Foot Shaoyang starts at the outer canthus. It ascends to the corner of the forehead and then winds downward to the back of the ear. The meridian descends along the lateral side of the neck in front of the Hand Shaoyang Meridian to the shoulder, where it crosses behind the Hand Shaoyang Meridian and enters the thoracic cavity through the supraclavicular fossa.

A branch of the Gallbladder Meridian splits off from the main course behind the ear and enters the ear. It then emerges in front of the ear and arrives at the outer canthus.

Another branch diverges from the main course at the outer canthus. It descends to the area anterior to the angle of the mandible, then winds upward to meet the Hand Shaoyang Meridian at the zygomatic region. From this point, the branch runs downward again to the angle of the mandible, passes along the lateral side of the neck, and briefly joins with the main course of the meridian at the supraclavicular fossa. The branch then descends into the chest, passes through the diaphragm, and connects with the liver and the gallbladder, the meridian's pertaining *fu* organ. It continues downward along the inside of the hypochondriac region and emerges from the inguinal region, passes downward around the margin of the pubic hair, and transversely enters the hip joint region.

Meanwhile, the main course of the meridian runs downward from the supraclavicular fossa along the surface of the trunk. It passes through the axilla, chest and hypochondriac region to the hip joint region, where it is rejoined by the branch. The main course then runs downward along the external side of the thigh and knee, and passes in front of the fibula on the leg. It then passes in front of the outer malleolus, goes along the lateral side of the top of the foot, and enters the interspace between the fourth and fifth toes.

The final branch of the meridian splits off from the main course at the top of the foot, goes obliquely to the big toe, and terminates at the medial side of the tip of the big toe.

If the meridian is diseased, there will be a bitter taste in the mouth, frequent sighing, pain in the precordial and hypochondriac regions aggravated by turning in bed; a slightly dusty facial complexion and rough, dry, dull skin in severe cases, and strephexopodia. All these conditions are due to yang reversal of the Foot Shaoyang Meridian.

The Gallbladder Meridian is indicated for treatment of disorders due to bone disturbance, including headache, pain below the lower jaw, pain at the outer canthus, swelling and pain in the supraclavicular fossa, swelling in the axillary region, lumps in the axillary region or below the lower jaw, sweating, chills, malaria, pain in the chest and side of the ribs; pain on the external side of the lower limb, pain in front of the outer malleolus, pain of all the joints, and motor impairment of the small toe.

12. Liver Meridian of Foot Jueyin

The Liver Meridian of Foot Jueyin originates at the hairy region on the top of the big toe. It runs upward along the top of the foot and ascends to the medial side of the leg 1 *cun* anterior to the inner malleolus. At 8 *cun* above the inner malleolus, the meridian crosses behind the Foot Taiyin Meridian. It runs upward along the medial side of the knee and the thigh to the pubic hair, and curves around the external genital region. The meridian then enters the abdominal cavity, passes upward alongside the stomach, and connects with the liver, its pertaining *zang* organ, and the gallbladder. Continuing upward within the cavity, it penetrates the diaphragm, distributes below the inside of the ribs, and follows the throat to the nasopharyngeal region. The meridian then ascends to connect with *muxi*, the tissues which connect the eyes with the brain, emerges from the forehead, and finally meets the Du Meridian on the top of the head [i.e. DU20-Baihui].

A branch of the Liver Meridian diverges from the main course at the eyes, descends to pass through the inside of the cheek, and encircles the inner surface of the lips.

Another branch splits off from the main course at the liver, ascends to penetrate the diaphragm, and pours into the lungs.

If the meridian is diseased, there will be lumbar pain aggravated by lying on the back or bending, swelling and pain of the testes in the male, lower abdominal pain and distension in the female, or even dry throat and a dull dusty facial complexion in severe cases.

The Liver Meridian is indicated for treatment of disorders due to liver dysfunction, including feeling of fullness in the chest, vomiting, hiccups, diarrhea with undigested food, inguinal hernia, nocturnal enuresis, and retention of urine.

Appendix 5

Pattern identification – deduce the invisible from the visible

The practice of acupuncture can be divided into four steps: pattern identification, principles of treatment, prescription, and puncture of acupoints ('the four Ps'). If the entire procedure is compared to a four-storey building, then pattern identification, *bian zheng* 辨证 in Chinese, is the ground floor. Patterns and pattern identification are fundamental to traditional Chinese medicine (TCM), and provide the basis for any treatment. Actual treatment is possible only if the practitioner can identify the pattern of a disease at each stage of its course (usually at the time of treatment).

There are many methods of pattern identification, each with its own characteristics. Within recent years many books have been published concerning specific methods of pattern identification. Here I will focus on some general questions concerning pattern identification as it relates to the clinical practice of acupuncture and related therapies.

Meaning and essential elements of patterns

Pattern is a translation of the Chinese medical term *zheng* 证, which literally means evidence or proof. Although there is no corresponding term in any other medical system, *zheng* is sometimes translated as syndrome, a term used in Western medicine to define a series of symptoms and signs, such as post-traumatic stress syndrome or premenstrual syndrome. However, there are substantial differences between pattern and syndrome, and it is incorrect to equate the two concepts.

There are numerous patterns, but each one is composed of only three basic elements – location, nature and time (formulated as $P = L + N + T$). Location refers to the position of the disease, and determines the target of treatment. Nature refers to the properties of the disease, and determines the specific principles of treatment. Time refers to the stage of the disease in each individual case.

For example, in the pattern known as flaming upward of the liver fire, the liver is the location of the disorder and excessive fire is its nature. Therefore, the liver is the target of treatment, and clearing liver fire is the principle of treatment. In the case of rebellious uprising of the stomach *qi*, the stomach is the location of the disorder and uprising of *qi* is its nature, so that the stomach is the target of treatment and the therapeutic principle is to subdue rebellious rising of the stomach *qi*. But where is the stage, or time factor in this overview of the condition? In fact, there is never one single time that can be identified. The course of a disease is a dynamic process in each individual case, and the pattern varies at different stages of its course, no matter whether the course is short or long.

Laws of patterns

Patterns are one of the most important concepts in traditional Chinese medicine. They adhere to the laws of invisibility, transformability, stability, simplicity and mutability.

Invisibility

Patterns are invisible. The pattern of each case reflects the essence of the disease or disorder at a particular stage of its course. It is always hidden among the numerous intricate and volatile manifestations that may arise. However, although the pattern is invisible, it can be grasped through its visible manifestations. Take flaming upward of the liver fire, for example. Excessive liver fire can be recognized through its manifestations, which include red eyes, flushed complexion, headache, irritability, yellow urine, red tongue with yellow coating, and wiry pulse. However, it is impossible actually to see the fire in the liver, even if the affected organ were to be surgically exposed. (See Figure A5.1.)

Transformability

Patterns are transformable. A disease undergoes a dynamic process in each individual case, and this process can be divided into a number of stages as the disease's pattern transforms over time. At each stage the disease remains the same, but both its location and

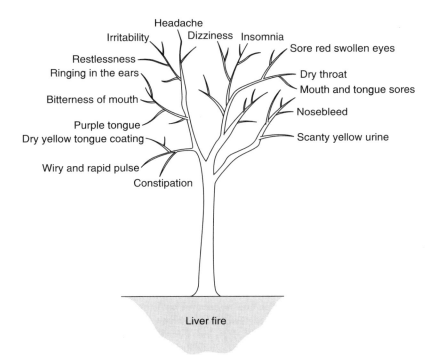

Figure A5.1 A life tree: the relation of pattern and manifestations. The Root represents the invisible pattern, and the Tips the visible manifestations.

nature may vary. Take stagnation of the liver *qi*, for example. Stagnant liver *qi* may transform into liver fire; the liver fire may then further consume the liver yin, or attack other internal organs such as the stomach, spleen, heart or lungs. Many factors may influence whether and how the pattern will transform, including the patient's constitution, the relative strength of the patient's right *qi* and evil *qi*, what treatment is given, the properties of the disease, etc. For example, if the patient possesses exuberant yang *qi* it is likely that the stagnant liver *qi* will transform into liver fire; while if the patient's stomach and spleen are deficient the stagnant liver *qi* will tend to attack these organs.

Stability
Patterns are stable in inverse relation to their transformability. Stability and transform-ability are two aspects of the whole, and cannot be separated. The properties of a disease influence the relative stability of its pattern. For instance, chronic conditions are more stable than acute problems. In some cases, the pattern of a chronic condition may remain unchanging for several or even many years, while the pattern of an acute disease may change from day to day.

Additionally, a pattern may be relatively stable even though its manifestations vary. For example, in a case of stagnation of the liver *qi* the patient may present various manifestations at different times, including a feeling of fullness in the chest, depression or restlessness, frequent sighing, headache, insomnia, dream-disturbed sleep, swollen and tender breasts, dysmenorrhea, etc. However, the pattern remains the same no matter how the manifestations change. Because patterns exhibit relative stability as well as transformability, it is possible to determine the pattern of a disease at any stage of its course.

Simplicity
Patterns are simple. Clinical manifestations are numerous and complicated, and sometimes contradictory, but patterns consist of clear and limited elements. Although patterns generally exhibit numerous manifestations, all patterns can be categorized according to the eight properties of yin, yang, exterior, interior, cold, heat, excess and deficiency. These properties are also ideal for categorizing a variety of clinical manifestations for ease of treatment.

Mutability
Patterns are mutable – that is, they change through time. Clinically, practitioners should always keep in mind that the pattern of each individual case may have changed since yesterday, and it may change again by tomorrow.

Differentiating pattern and manifestations

A pattern consists of a series of manifestations. The pattern reflects a condition's interior, invisible essence at a particular stage of its course, while manifestations are the condition's exterior, visible appearance. A pattern is like the roots of a tree, which lie hidden deep within the earth. Manifestations are the tips of the tree, above ground and visible for all to see. (See Figure A5.1.) The invisible pattern can be identified by analyzing and synthesizing its visible manifestations. The purpose of treatment is permanently to sever the Root of the condition (the pattern), rather than temporarily to cut back its Tip (the manifestations).

Differentiating pattern and disease

One disease, many patterns
As mentioned above, a disease is a dynamic process. Each individual case can be divided into a number of stages, according to the pattern it is currently manifesting. In other words, one case of a disease may exhibit many different patterns. Proper treatment must be applied at each stage of the disease, according to pattern. This is the reason that various treatments may be applied during the course of one case of a disease.

Same disease, different patterns
People who are considered to have the same disease in terms of modern medicine may exhibit different patterns due to differences in constitution, sex, age, etc. For example, two patients suffer from the common cold. One of them may have severe chills, no fever or sweating, headache, stiff neck, a thin whitish tongue coating and a floating and tense pulse, while the other may have high fever, mild chills, sweating, a sore throat, a thin yellow tongue coating and a floating and rapid pulse. Although they have the same disease, their patterns are opposite. The first exhibits wind-cold pattern of the common cold, and the second wind-heat pattern of the common cold. As their patterns are different, so their treatments should be different as well. The principle of treatment in the first case is to expel wind-cold, while in the second case it is to clear heat. This is the reason that different treatments may be used for different cases of the same disease.

Different disease, same pattern
This situation is the opposite of the previous one. People who are considered to have different diseases in terms of modern medicine may exhibit the same pattern at a particular stage. For example, stagnation of liver *qi* is a common pattern of a number of disorders, including headache, hysteria, neurosis, sexual dysfunction, premenstrual syndrome and dysmenorrhea. If patients with any of these disorders are found to be experiencing stagnation of liver *qi* at a particular stage of their illness, they can be cured using the same treatment. This is the reason that the same treatment may be used for different diseases.

Pattern identification and Root and Tip theory

As discussed in Chapter 1, the concept of Root and Tip is as important to Chinese philosophy and traditional Chinese medicine as that of Yin and Yang. Root and Tip theory is an integral part of pattern identification.

The principle of Yin and Yang brings to light the universal law of the unity of opposites, while the principle of Root and Tip reveals the specific law of the difference between opposites. Root refers to the principal aspect of two opposites or a contradiction, while Tip is the secondary aspect of two opposites or a contradiction. Like the relationship between the root of a tree and its tips, the principal aspect of two opposites or a contradiction occupies the leading place and determines the onset and development of the secondary aspect. To solve a problem, it is essential to distinguish the principal from the secondary. Once the principal aspect of two opposites or a contradiction is dealt with, the secondary aspect may disappear simultaneously or be solved with ease.

When human beings are in a state of good health, the body's yin and yang are in balance. These two aspects of the whole are equivalent, and neither is principal or secondary. However, when disharmony occurs a contradiction arises between the body's yin and yang and they can be categorized in terms of Root and Tip. Take deficiency of yin *qi*, for example. In this case, the body's yin *qi* is insufficient, but the yang *qi* is normal. Therefore, deficiency of yin *qi* is the Root or principal aspect of the pattern, and the therapeutic principle is that the yin *qi* should be nourished.

The following four primary Root and Tip pairs are utilized in pattern identification.

Right qi *and evil* qi

Right *qi*, *zheng qi* in Chinese, refers to the materials or functions of the body that defend against invasion by pathogens. Evil *qi*, *xie qi* in Chinese, refers to pathogenic factors which may lead to illnesses. Root represents right *qi* and Tip refers to evil *qi*. In this case, the struggle of these two entities decides the onset, development and prognosis of a disease. If the right *qi* is strong enough, no disease will occur. Disease is an indication that the right *qi* is insufficient.

In general, diseases can be divided into excessive and deficient according to the relative strength of right *qi* and evil *qi*. Excessive patterns are pathological conditions in which the evil *qi* (or pathogenic factor) is hyperactive, but there is sufficient right *qi* to contend with it. Deficient patterns are pathological conditions in which, although there are no pathogenic factors, there is insufficient right *qi* to maintain health. The *Neijing* states: 'Hyperactivity of evil *qi* causes excess; consumption of right *qi* leads to deficiency'[1].

Etiology and disease

Etiology and disease refer simply to the cause and effect of imbalance. Etiology (the Root) encompasses the factors that result in disease (the Tip). In this case, Root and Tip have a direct causal relationship. For example, anger (the Root) may result in stagnation of the liver *qi* (the Tip), or overeating may be the cause of retention of food in the stomach. After onset of the disease, the cause may either persist or disappear. For example, the emotional factor of anger may exist throughout the course of the problem, while the act of overeating may stop when there is retention of food in the stomach. In many cases, the cause of a condition can be ascertained through inquiry.

Pathogenesis and clinical manifestations

Pathogenesis refers to the location and nature of a pattern. In this case, Root and Tip are not separate entities but a unity. Pathogenesis, or essence, is the Root of the pattern, and the clinical manifestations, or appearance, are its Tip. Root and Tip, pathogenesis and clinical manifestations, essence and appearance – these pairs reflect the two aspects of the pattern, and are inseparably related to each other. They have the following relationships:

1. *Exterior and interior.* Clinical manifestations are exterior and can be detected through examination, while pathogenesis is interior and can only be grasped through abstract analysis. For example, the clinical manifestations of flaming upward of the stomach fire, such as a flushed facial complexion and reddened tongue with a yellow dry coating, are detectable. However, it would be futile to attempt to see whether or not there is fire in the stomach. This relation is the same as that between the fall of an apple and gravity. Anyone can see an apple fall, but not even Newton could actually see gravity.

2. *General and specific.* Pathogenesis represents the general condition, while the related clinical manifestations reflect its specific aspects. That is, one pathogenesis may have various manifestations, and a number of manifestations may share one pathogenesis. For example, flaming upward of the liver fire may manifest as headache, tinnitus, redness of the eyes, bitter taste in the mouth, dry throat, restlessness, irritability, flushed facial complexion, a reddened tongue with yellow coating and a wiry and rapid pulse, while each of these manifestations is a reflection of the underlying pathogenesis.
3. *Stability and changeability.* Pathogenesis is relatively stable, while clinical manifestations are changeable. During the course of a disease or disorder, the pathogenesis may remain the same even though its clinical manifestations decrease or increase. For example, people with Shaoyang Pattern of the common cold may exhibit different manifestations at different stages, such as alternating chills and fever on the first day and bitter taste in the mouth and vomiting the next, but the pathogenesis, or essence of the pattern, remains the same.

The relationship between pathogenesis (Root) and clinical manifestations (Tip), which is non-causal, may easily be confused with the relationship between etiology (Root) and disease (Tip), which is causal. However, it is completely wrong to consider pathogenesis to be the cause of a condition's clinical manifestations; rather, pathogenesis and clinical manifestations are two inter-related aspects of the overall condition. Clinical manifestations (appearance) are signals that pathology exists, while pathogenesis (essence) identifies specific components of the pathology.

Initial onset and subsequent diseases or patterns
Clinical cases are usually complex rather than simple, and this means that there are often two or more kinds of diseases or patterns coexisting simultaneously. In terms of time, the disease or pattern that occurs first is considered to be the Root, while subsequent developments are considered the Tip. In this case Root and Tip are two entities, which may have either a causal or non-causal relationship. In the case of a causal relationship, the initial (or Root) disease or pattern is the cause of subsequent (or Tip) diseases or patterns. For instance, in case of invasion of the stomach by hyperactive liver *qi*, hyperactive liver *qi* is the initial pattern and the cause of the subsequent stomach disorder. In the case of a non-causal relationship, the initial (or Root) disease or pattern and subsequent (or Tip) diseases or patterns occur in sequence. For example, if a person with chronic cough has a sudden trauma, there is no relationship between the initial cough and the subsequent trauma.

The concept of Root and Tip is very useful for identifying patterns. The four Root and Tip pairs discussed above are all important for pattern identification, particularly pathogenesis and clinical manifestations. The task of pattern identification can be generalized into distinguishing the Root from the Tip. It is particularly important to identify the Root of a condition. The *Neijing* summarizes: 'To treat the disease one must seek the root'[2].

Procedure of pattern identification

Pattern identification is a comprehensive process of applying all the basic theories of traditional Chinese medicine. There are various methods, each with its own characteristics. Generally speaking, the complete process of pattern identification can be divided into the following five steps.

Step 1: determine the position of the disease at a particular stage
It is necessary to locate the position of a disease at each stage of its course, because the position of the disease is the target of treatment. According to traditional Chinese medicine, the human body consists of two systems: the *zangfu* organ system and the meridian system. Locating the position of a disease therefore involves determining which organ or meridian is being affected.

For example, headache is a common symptom. The head is the location of the symptom, but the position of the disease may vary in different conditions, depending on which meridians or *zangfu* organs are affected. If the headache is due to flaming upward of the liver fire, the liver will be the position of disease; if it is due to flaming upward of the stomach fire, the stomach will be the position of disease.

It is also necessary to make a distinction between the position of a disease according to traditional Chinese medicine and that according to modern medicine. For instance, in terms of modern medicine the subcortex is the position of the disease neurosis, but according to traditional Chinese medicine various organs might be involved, including the liver, heart, kidney, stomach, spleen and gallbladder.

Locating the position of the disease is of primary importance in pattern identification. The position of a disease is the target, and subsequent treatment is the arrow. Only if the target is correctly determined can the arrow be shot accurately. Otherwise, the effort will be futile no matter how skillful the practitioner is.

The following methods are used to determine the position of a disease:

1. Zangfu *theory.* According to *zangfu* theory, the human body consists of five subsystems (i.e. liver, heart, spleen, lung and kidney.) The five *zang* organs are the core of these subsystems. Each subsystem has a corresponding *fu* organ, and is associated with a particular element, color, taste, sensory organ, body tissue and emotion. (See Table A5.1.) Pathologically, the internal *zangfu* organs are considered to be the position of diseases of both the organs themselves, and their associated sensory organs and tissues. For example, the liver opens into the eyes, so the liver is considered to be the position of disease of various eye problems, such as glaucoma and hysteric blindness. Similarly, the lungs function to nourish the skin, so the lungs are considered to be the position of disease of various skin problems.
2. *Meridian theory.* The meridians form an interconnected network throughout the body. This network consists primarily of the twelve Regular Meridians and the Ren and Du Meridians, known as the Fourteen Meridians. Each meridian has its own pathway and connections. According to meridian theory, the position of a disease is considered to be the meridian along whose pathway or connections it occurs. For example, the Lung Meridian connects internally with the lung, large intestine, trachea and cardia; externally it connects with the throat and runs along the supraclavicular fossa and anterior border of the medial aspect of the upper limb. Therefore, the Lung Meridian is considered to be the position of disease of any disorders that occur along its pathway or in its connecting organs, including cough, asthma, shortness of breath, pain or feeling of fullness in the chest, hemoptysis, swelling and pain in the throat, pain in the supraclavicular fossa, shoulder pain that is aggravated by abduction, and pain, numbness or any skin problem along its pathway on the upper limb.
3. *Tongue and pulse examination.* The appearance of the tongue and the condition of the pulse are important signs in pattern identification. They are used to determine both the position and the nature of disease. In the clinic it is sometimes possible to establish a diagnosis just by looking at the patient's tongue[3].

Table A5.1
Some associations of the five *zang* organs

Zang organ	Element	*Fu* organ	Color	Taste	Sensory organ	Tissue	Emotion
Liver	Wood	Gallbladder	Gray	Sour	Eyes	Tendons	Anger
Heart	Fire	Small intestine	Red	Bitter	Tongue	Blood vessels	Joy
Spleen	Earth	Stomach	Yellow	Sweet	Mouth	Muscle	Meditation
Lung	Metal	Large intestine	White	Pungent	Nose	Skin and hair	Grief
Kidney	Water	Urinary bladder	Black	Salty	Ears	Bone	Fear

4. *Etiology.* The etiology or cause of disease can often be determined by asking patients about the onset of the condition, their lifestyle, and their living and working environment. A complete understanding of the cause of a disease is helpful in locating its position. For example, exogenous wind-cold tends first to invade the Lung and Urinary Bladder Meridians, improper diet damages the stomach and spleen, anger hurts the liver, and excessive sexual activity consumes the kidney essence.

To summarize, the position of disease can be clarified using *zangfu* theory, meridian theory, tongue and pulse examination, and etiology. Although it is often possible to determine the position of disease using only one or two methods, it is recommended to make full use of all of them in order to avoid mistakes and be assured of a correct target.

Step 2: determine the nature of the disease at a particular stage of its course

Determining the nature of a disease involves identifying its properties at a particular stage of its course. The nature of a disease determines how it will be treated. Although clinical manifestations are numerous, complicated and sometimes even contradictory, the nature of all diseases can be categorized in terms of the following general properties: yin and yang, exterior and interior, cold and heat (or fire), excess and deficiency, *qi*, blood, wind, dampness and dryness, and phlegm. Some common conditions are yin or yang deficiency, stagnation of *qi*, exterior wind-cold, interior damp-heat, etc.

The following elements are used to determine the nature of a disease:

1. *Symptoms.* Many clinical symptoms can clearly and definitively indicate the nature of a disease. For example, chills indicate exterior wind-cold; low tolerance for cold and cold limbs is a typical manifestation of yang deficiency; stabbing pain indicates stagnant blood; distending pain indicates stagnation of *qi*; and dull pain indicates insufficiency of *qi*, blood or essence.
2. *Signs.* The appearance of the tongue and the condition of the pulse are valuable in determining the nature of a disease. For example, a purple tongue indicates stagnant blood; a pale tongue indicates deficient *qi* and/or blood; a thick, dry, yellow tongue coating indicates excessive fire; a thready pulse indicates yin deficiency; and a wiry pulse indicates stagnation of the liver *qi*.
3. *Etiology.* A complete understanding of the causes of a disease is useful in determining its nature. For instance, exogenous pathogens usually result in excessive conditions; people who live or work in damp surroundings over long periods may suffer from dampness; longstanding emotional injury may lead to stagnation of *qi* and blood; and excessive sexual activity consumes the kidney essence, resulting in deficient conditions.

4. *The properties of disease in terms of modern medicine.* The properties of disease in terms of modern medicine (i.e. acute, chronic, infectious, depressive, excitative, etc.) are closely related to its nature at a certain stage of its course. For instance, infectious diseases such as tonsillitis and conjunctivitis involve excessive heat; hypotension indicates deficiency of *qi* and blood; and hypertension is usually excessive in Tip and deficient in Root.
5. *Others.* In general, chronic problems are deficient and acute problems are excessive. Patients who are in generally good health tend to have excessive conditions, while those in poor health usually manifest deficient conditions.

When determining the nature of a disease, it is important not to confuse nature with etiology, especially in the case of exogenous conditions. Etiology and disease have a causal relationship, while nature and disease exhibit the unified relationship of essence and appearance[4]. Take heat pattern, for example. If heat pattern is induced by external heat pathogens, both the etiology of the disease (external heat pathogens) and the nature of the disease are heat.

However, heat pattern can also be the result of invasion of the body by external cold pathogens. In this case, the etiology of the disease (cold pathogens) is cold, while the nature of the disease is heat.

Step 3: combine the position and nature of the disease
Locating the position of a disease establishes the target of treatment, and identifying its nature determines the principles to be used in selecting treatment. The pattern is identified by combining these two factors.

For instance, if the liver is the position of the disease and stagnant *qi* is its nature, the pattern may be identified as stagnation of liver *qi*. Consequently, the liver is the target of treatment and the therapeutic principle is to promote the flow of liver *qi*. In the same way, if the stomach is the position of the disease and retention of food is its nature, the pattern will be identified as retention of food in the stomach, with the stomach as the target of treatment and the therapeutic principle to stimulate the stomach in order to remove the retained food.

The ongoing process of pattern identification could be terminated and treatment implemented in the two examples mentioned above. However, the majority of cases are by no means so simple. On the one hand, as mentioned above, each case of a disease is a dynamic process. Both the position and nature of the disease will change during the course of an illness, no matter whether the course is short or long. On the other hand, the patterns commonly seen in practice are generally complex rather than simple. They may include simultaneous disorders of the exterior and the interior, or combined cold-heat or excess-deficiency conditions. It is therefore necessary to undertake the following two steps.

Step 4: grasp the transformation rules of patterns
As mentioned above, the position of a disease may shift and its nature may transform throughout its course. If either or both of these factors change, the pattern will change as well, requiring alterations in treatment. Although pattern transformations are various and complicated, they follow a number of rules. The position of a disease may shift in the following ways:

1. *Shifts among the* zangfu *organs.* The human body is an organic whole, and the closed relationship among the *zangfu* organs can be defined from the following perspectives.

- ☙ Through the meridians. The five primary *zang* organs are connected internally and externally with the five *fu* organs through the meridians. The *zang* and *fu* organs support each other physiologically, while pathologically they may mutually affect each other. For example, the stomach and spleen are exterior–interior related. Normally, the stomach governs the intake and metabolism of water and food, and the spleen governs the movement and transformation of water and food. Pathologically, they may affect each other and lead to deficiency of the stomach and spleen.
- ☙ According to Five Elements theory. The five *zang* organs are each associated with one of the Five Elements, which are considered to engender each other in the following order: wood gives birth to fire, fire gives birth to earth, earth gives birth to metal, metal gives birth to water, and water gives birth to wood. Based on this correspondence, the *zang* organs engender each other in the following order: liver (wood), heart (fire), spleen (earth), lungs (metal) and kidneys (water). This is referred to as the Mother–Child relationship. Each organ is the Child of the organ that engenders it, and the Mother of the organ it engenders. For example, the liver (wood) is the Child of the kidneys (water) and the Mother of the heart (fire) (i.e. wood is engendered by water, and gives birth to fire). Pathologically, disorder of an organ may disturb both its Mother and Child. For instance, dysfunction of the liver may affect the heart and/or invade the kidneys.
- ☙ Finally, according to Five Elements theory, the five *zang* organs exert a mutually regulating effect which prevents any of them becoming hyperactive. They control each other in the order of liver (wood), spleen (earth), kidneys (water), heart (fire) and lungs (metal). Pathologically, if any of the *zang* organs is excessive or deficient, the related organs will be involved and the balance will be upset. The *Neijing* states: 'When a *zang* organ is in excess, it will overwhelm the organ it controls and rise in rebellion against the organ which controls it; when a *zang* organ is in deficiency, it will be overwhelmed by the organ which controls it and be bullied by the organ it controls'[5]. For example, the liver (wood) normally controls the spleen (earth) and is controlled by the lungs (metal). If the liver *qi* is hyperactive, it will overwhelm the spleen and insult the lungs, while if the liver *qi* is deficient, it will be overwhelmed by the lungs and insulted by the spleen.

2. *Shifts among the meridians.* The meridians connect the upper with the lower and the interior with the exterior, joining the body into an organic whole. Normally, the meridians serve as channels for the flow of *qi* and blood, while pathologically they are pathways for the transmission of pathogens. Pathogens may be transmitted through the meridians in two ways:

   - ☙ There may be transmission between the related interior–exterior meridians. Because they are so closely related, disturbance of a meridian may shift to its interior–exterior related meridian with ease. For example, the Kidney and Urinary Bladder Meridians are interior–exterior related. If exogenous wind-cold invades the Urinary Bladder Meridian, it may easily shift into the Kidney Meridian.
   - ☙ There may be transmission among the six Foot Meridians. This phenomenon is seen in cases of cold-induced disease, and is discussed in detail in the *Neijing* and *Discussion on Cold Induced Diseases*[6].

3. *Shifts from the meridians to the* zangfu *organs or* vice versa. The twelve Regular Meridians connect internally with the *zangfu* organs and externally with the various tissues of the body. Normally the meridians and *zangfu* organs cooperate with each

other, while pathologically they mutually affect each other. For example, disturbance of the Urinary Bladder Meridian by wind-cold may affect the function of the urinary bladder and lead to difficulty in urination. This is also known as transmission from the exterior to the interior. Conversely, when the urinary bladder is out of order, there may be manifestations such as pain and coldness along the external pathway of its meridian. This is known as transmission from the interior to the exterior.

Changes in the nature of a disease also follow a number of rules. Excessive yang may consume yin fluid and lead to yin deficiency; excessive yin may damage yang *qi* and lead to yang deficiency. An excess of pathogens may injure right *qi* and lead to deficient conditions. Excessive cold may cause yang *qi* to stagnate, and the stagnant yang *qi* may then lead to excessive heat; while excessive heat may force profuse fluid out of the body and lead to deficient cold. Stagnant *qi* may either transform into fire or lead to stagnation of the blood. Deficiency of blood may either lead to stagnation of the blood, or engender endogenous wind. Extreme heat will consume the body fluid and will also produce endogenous wind. Longstanding accumulation of dampness may condense into sticky phlegm.

The position and nature of a disease may change either separately or simultaneously. In some cases the position of a disease changes but its nature stays the same, while in others the position remains fixed but the nature changes. Regardless of which changes, the pattern will be transformed. Various factors influence the transformation of a pattern, including the relative strength of right *qi* and evil *qi*, method of treatment, exercise, rest, diet, lifestyle and state of mind. If a patient has strong right *qi* and weak pathogens, receives appropriate treatment, gets proper activity and rest and an adequate diet, and has a positive outlook, the condition will take a favorable turn. Otherwise, the reverse may be the case. In addition to implementing timely and effective treatment, it is therefore necessary to increase all favorable factors and decrease any unfavorable ones in order to improve the condition.

Step 5: make a clear distinction between Root and Tip
Making a clear distinction between Root and Tip has two purposes. In the narrow sense, it serves to identify initial (Root) and subsequent (Tip) conditions. Clinically, many cases are complex rather than simple. For instance, chronic and acute or interior and exterior conditions may be present at the same time. The relation between initial and subsequent conditions may be causal or not, and it is very important to determine this relationship in order to formulate correct therapeutic principles. If the relationship is causal both the initial and subsequent conditions should be treated, otherwise the subsequent condition may easily recur even after being temporarily cured. For example, patients with chronic lung disease are susceptible to catching cold, so their chronic lung problem should also be treated in order to avoid frequent recurrence of the common cold. If the relationship between Root and Tip conditions is not causal, they may be treated either simultaneously or separately in order of urgency.

In the broader sense, distinguishing between Root and Tip is the final synthesis of the first four steps of pattern identification – locating the position of the disease, determining its nature, combining its position and nature, and grasping the rules of transformation. Each of these steps utilizes the concept of Root and Tip to clarify different aspects of the condition. In practice, the four steps are often not a sequential, orderly process, but are rather woven together. The final step of distinguishing Root and Tip makes it possible to systematize all results in order to attribute a clear and definite pattern to a condition at a particular stage of its course. (See Table A5.2.) Once the Root of a condition is recognized

Table A5.2
Summary of Root and Tip pairs used in pattern identification and steps in which they are used

Step	*Root*	*Tip*	*Relation between Root and Tip*
Step 2: determine nature of the disease	Right *qi*	Evil *qi*	Opposites
Step 2: determine nature of the disease	Cause	Disease	Cause and effect
Steps 1 and 2: determine position and nature of the disease	Pathogenesis (location and nature)	Clinical manifestations	Essence and appearance
Steps 4 and 5: grasp rules of transformation, distinguish between Root and Tip	Initial onset	Subsequent onset	Cause and effect or unrelated

it is possible to determine the appropriate therapeutic principle and, because the Root is primary, treating the Root alone will often be sufficient to achieve a cure.

Unfortunately, the importance of the concept of Root and Tip often tends to be overlooked in practice. The *Neijing* states[7]:

> Understanding the principle of Root and Tip aids one in treatment; not understanding it is a virtual blindness in treatment . . . The principle of Root and Tip is simple, yet clinically it is quite difficult to grasp.

Differences in pattern identification in acupuncture and herbal medicine
Both acupuncture and herbal medicine are based on the fundamental theories of traditional Chinese medicine. However, there are major differences in how the two healing methods approach pattern identification.

Locating the position of the disease is of primary importance in acupuncture treatment. As discussed in Chapter 3, the effects of a meridian's acupoints are dependent primarily on the connections established by the meridian. Therefore, when prescribing acupoints it is necessary to identify which meridian is affected. For instance, in a case of frozen shoulder, the position of disease may be the Lung, Large Intestine, San Jiao or Small Intestine Meridians. Acupoints are prescribed according to the specifically affected meridians, regardless of differences in the nature of the disease. Herbal medicine, however, gives priority to the nature rather than the position of the disease. Although medicinal herbs are considered to affect specific meridians, they are prescribed according to the specific nature of the disease, regardless of differences in the position of the disease.

Identification of the nature of a disease is much more important in herbal medicine than in acupuncture. Medications, both modern and traditional, have unidirectional effects. A cold herb is always cold; it can never also be warm. Correctly determining the nature of the disease is therefore crucial when prescribing herbs. For instance, if cold herbs are used for a pattern with a cold nature, the condition will become worse. This is not necessarily true in the case of acupuncture, thanks to the bi-directional beneficial effect of acupoints. Puncturing the same acupoint can cure patterns with opposite natures. As long as the position of the disease is correctly determined and the correct acupoint stimulated, the body itself will harmonize the condition automatically.

Of course, emphasizing the importance of locating the position of the disease in acupuncture treatment does not mean that it is not necessary to determine the nature of the disease. It is true that for general conditions there may be no adverse effects, and there may even be improvement, if treatment is carried out when the nature of the condition is unknown. However, it cannot be overemphasized that it is crucial to apply proper treatment in extreme conditions. Particularly in cases of severely excessive or deficient conditions, improper needling stimulation may lead to serious adverse effects.

Notes and references

1. *Suwen*, 28:173.
2. *Suwen*, 5:31.
3. I once treated a patient with severe headache. The pain was so severe that he sometimes even lost consciousness. The patient had been treated with modern medicine, and the doctors thought that something was wrong inside his head. As soon as I had a look at his tongue, I had an idea what was happening. The tongue coating was thick, dry, and burned yellow. It is well known that this type of tongue coating usually indicates excessive stomach fire. This inference was verified by inquiry. The patient stated that he had not defecated in over 2 weeks (it was very strange that he had no discomfort in the abdomen). A prescription of four herbs was given to loosen the bowels and cool heat. (This method is known as 'raking firewood from beneath the cauldron in order to stop boiling'.) Two hours after taking the herbs he had a bowel movement with a dark and bloody stool, and the headache miraculously disappeared.
4. Westerners often confuse the causal relationship of etiology and disease with the non-causal relationship of nature and disease. Ted J. Kaptchuk writes:

   > Chinese medicine and Chinese philosophy, as we have seen, do not concern themselves very much with cause and effect, or with trying to discover this cause that begets, in linear progression, that effect. Their concern is with relationships, with the pattern of events. Thus, their idea of the way illness begins is very different from the Western view.
   >
   > In fact, the Chinese do not have a highly developed theory for the origins of disease. They conceive of certain factors that affect the body, factors that could be described in the Western vocabulary as causes. It is therefore tempting to the Western mind to describe them as such, but to the Chinese these generative factors are not exactly causes. Take dampness, for example. In China, as in the West, people might say that someone became ill because he or she went out in the rain or got his feet muddy or because he lives in a damp basement. But to the Chinese, dampness precipitates only a pattern of Dampness; there is no distinction between the illness itself and the factor that 'caused' it. The question of cause becomes incidental. In this sense, the word *cause* is almost a synonym for *effect*. Dampness is recognized by what is going on inside, not by knowledge of external exposure. The condition is not *caused* by Dampness; the condition is Dampness. The cause is the effect; the line is a circle. From Ted J. Kaptchuk, *Chinese Medicine – The Web that has no Weaver*. London: Rider, 1983, 115–117.

5. *Suwen*, 67:386.
6. On the first day of *shanghan* or invasion of the body by exogenous cold, the Urinary Bladder Meridian of Foot Taiyang is attacked. As the meridian distributes on the head, back of the neck, and back, so one will manifest headache, stiff neck, and ache in the back. On the second day, the pathogen is transferred to the Stomach Meridian of Foot Yangming. This meridian controls musculature and connects with the nose and eyes. Therefore the symptoms will manifest as fever, pain in the eyes, dry nose, and difficulty lying in any position. On the third day, the disease progresses to the Gallbladder Meridian of Foot Shaoyang. This meridian passes through the bilateral rib areas and connects with the ears, so there will be pain in the rib region and deafness. . . . On the fourth day, the pathogen is transferred to the Spleen Meridian of Foot Taiyin. This

meridian connects with the stomach and throat, so there will be abdominal distention and dry throat. On the fifth day, the disease progresses to the Kidney Meridian of Foot Shaoyin. This meridian connects with the kidneys, lungs, and the root of the tongue, so the patient may have thirst and dryness of the mouth and tongue. On the sixth day, the pathogen travels to the Liver Meridian of Foot Jueyin. This meridian goes along the external genital region and connects with the liver, so there will be restlessness, feeling of fullness in the chest, and contraction of the scrotum. *Suwen*, 31:183.

7. *Suwen*, 65:356.

Bibliography

References in Chinese (classical)

Collation and Annotation of the Lingshu (*Lingshujing Jiaoshi* 灵枢经校释) (*c*. 104–32 BC) (ed. Hebei Medical College *et al*.). Beijing: People's Health Press, 1984. This annotation is based on the version of the *Lingshu* published by the Jujingtang Printing House (居敬堂) during the Ming Dynasty (1522–1566 AD).

Collation and Annotation of the Suwen (*Huang Di Neijing Suwen Jiaoshi* 黄帝内经素问校释) (*c*. 104–32 BC) (ed. Shandong College of Traditional Chinese Medicine *et al*.). Beijing: People's Health Press, 1982. This annotation is based on the version of the *Suwen* annotated by Lin Yi (ed. 1056–1067 AD) and Gu Congde (ed. 1550 AD).

Compilation and Annotation of the Yellow Emperor's Classic of Bright Halls (*Huang Di Mingtangjing Jijiao* 黄帝明堂经辑校) (*c*. 32 BC–106 AD.) (ed. Huang Longxiang (contemporary)). Beijing: Chinese Medicine and Science Press, 1987.

Collation and Annotation of the Book of Meridians from Zhangjiashan (*Zhangjiashan Hanjian Maishu Jiaoshi* 张家山汉简脉书校释) (ed. Gao Dalun (contemporary)). Chengdu: Chengdu Press, 1992.

Guanzi (*Guanzi* 管子). Beijing: Yanshan Press, 1995. The *Guanzi* is a collection of the ideas of Guanzi (*c*. 725–645 BC) and his followers, compiled during the Warring States Period (475–221 BC).

Huangfu Mi (*c*. 215–282 AD), *Systematic Classic of Acupuncture and Moxibustion*, also translated as *ABC of Acupuncture and Moxibustion* (*Zhenjiu Jiayijing* 针灸甲乙经) (*c*. 256–259 AD) (ed. Huang Longxiang (contemporary)). Beijing: Chinese Medicine and Science Press, 1990.

Huainanzi (*Huainanzi* 淮南子) (*c*. Western Han Dynasty, 206 BC–24 AD). Beijing: Yanshan Press, 1995.

Laozi: Annotation and Appreciation of Laozi (*Laozi Zhushi Ji Pingjie* 老子注释及评介) (ed. Chen Guying (contemporary)). Beijing: China Book Company, 1984. Based on the *Laozi* (*Daodejing* 道德经), a collection of the ideas of Laozi (*c*. sixth century BC) and his followers, compiled during the early Warring States Period (475–221 BC).

Lingshu – the Spiritual Pivot (*Lingshujing* 灵枢经) (*c*. 104–32 BC). Beijing: People's Health Press, 1963. The *Lingshu* is the earlier part of the *The Yellow Emperor's Inner Classic of Medicine* or *The Neijing* (*Huang Di Neijing* 黄帝内经) (*c*. 104–32 BC), the seminal work of traditional Chinese medicine. This version of the *Lingshu* was first published by the Jujingtang Printing House (居敬堂) during the Ming Dynasty (1522–1566 AD). It is the version quoted in this book.

Li Shizhen (1518–1593 AD), *A Study on the Eight Extraordinary Meridians* (*Qijing Bamai Kao* 奇经八脉考) (1578 AD). Shanghai: Shanghai Science and Technology Publishing House, 1990.

Ma Jixing (contemporary), *Study and Annotation of the Ancient Medical Relics of Mawangdui* (*Mawangdui Guyishu Kaoshi* 马王堆古医书考释). Hunan: Hunan Science and Technology Press, 1992.

Nanjing – the Classic of Difficulties (*Nanjing* 难经) (*c*. prior to 25 AD). Beijing: Scientific and Technological Documents Publishing House, 1996.

Sima Qian (*c*. 135 BC–?), *The Historical Records* (*Shi Ji* 史记) (*c*. 100 BC) (ed. Liu Xinglin *et al*.). Beijing: China Friendship Publishing Company, 1994.

Suwen – The Simple Questions: The Inner Classic of the Yellow Emperor (*Huang Di Neijing Suwen* 黄帝内经素问) (*c*. 104–32 BC), annotated by Wang Bing, 762 AD. Beijing: People's Health Press, 1963. The *Suwen* is the later part of the *Neijing – The Yellow Emperor's Classic of Medicine* (*Huang Di Neijing*) (*c*. 104–32 BC), the seminal work of traditional Chinese medicine. This is the version of the *Suwen* quoted in this book.

Wang Weiyi (987–1067 AD), *Illustrated Classic of Acupoints on the Bronze Model* (*Tongren Shuxue Zhenjiu Tujing* 铜人腧穴针灸图经) (1027 AD). Beijing: China Bookstore, 1987.

Xu Feng (*c*. Ming Dynasty, 1368–1644 AD), *Complete Book of Acupuncture and Moxibustion* (*Zhenjiu Daquan* 针灸大全) (1439 AD). Beijing: People's Health Press, 1987.

Yang Jizhou (1522–1619 AD), *Compendium of Acupuncture and Moxibustion* (*Zhenjiu Dacheng* 针灸大成) (1601 AD). Beijing: People's Health Press, 1963.

Yang Shangshan (*c*. 610–682 AD), *The Yellow Emperor's Inner Classic of Medicine: the Great Simplicity* (*Huang Di Neijing Taisu* 黄帝内经太素) (*c*. 650 AD). Beijing: People's Health Press, 1965. This is the earliest extant annotation of the *Neijing*, including both the *Lingshu* and the *Suwen*. Twenty-three of the thirty original chapters are extant.

Zhang Zhongjing (*c*. 150–219 AD), *Discussion of Cold Induced Diseases* (*Shanghan Lun* 伤寒论) (*c*. 200–210 AD). Beijing: People's Health Press, 1976.

Zhuangzi: Brief Annotations of Zhuangzi (*Zhuangzi Qianzhu* 庄子浅注) (ed. Cao Chuji (contemporary)). Beijing: China Book Company, 1982. Based on the *Zhuangzi* (*Zhuangzi* 庄子), a collection of the ideas of Zhuangzi (*c*. 369–286 BC) and his followers, compiled during the late Warring States Period (475–221 AD).

References in Chinese (modern)

Guo Shiyu, *The History of Chinese Acupuncture and Moxibustion* (*Zhongguo Zhenjiu Shi* 中国针灸史). Tianjin: Tianjin Science and Technology Press, 1989.

He Puren, *Acupuncture Needling Methods* (*Zhenju Zhenfa* 针具针法). Beijing: Scientific and Technical Documents Publishing House, 1989.

He Puren, *Relief of Pain with Acupuncture* (*Zhenjiu Zhitong* 针灸治痛). Beijing: Scientific and Technical Documents Publishing House, 1995.

Li Ding *et al*., *Meridian Theory* (*Jingluo Xue* 经络学). Shanghai: Shanghai Science and Technology Press, 1984.

Li Shizhen, *Discussion on the Utilization of Commonly Used Acupuncture Points* (*Changyong Shuxue Linchuang Fahui* 常用腧穴临床发挥). Beijing: People's Health

Press, 1985. (This contemporary author should not be confused with the classical Li Shizhen (1518–1593 AD) mentioned above.)

Li Zhicao *et al.*, *Mystery of Thousands of Years – Research on the Physical Properties of the Meridians* (*Qiangu Zhi Mi – Jingluo Wuli Texing Yanjiu* 千古之谜—经络物理特性研究). Chengdu: Sichuan Education Press, 1988.

Lu Jingshan *et al.*, *A Collection of Treatments Using One Acupoint* (*Danxue Zhibing Xuancui* 单穴治病选粹). Beijing: People's Health Press, 1993.

Ren Jiyu, *History of Chinese Philosophy* (*Zhongguo Zhexue Shi* 中国哲学史). Beijing: People's Press, 1966.

Tang De'an *et al.*, *Experimental Acupuncture and Moxibustion* (*Shiyan Zhenjiu Xue* 实验针灸学). Tianjin: Publishing House of Tianjin College of Traditional Chinese Medicine, 1983.

Wang Benxian, *Foreign Research on the Meridians* (*Guowai Dui Jingluo Wenti De Yanjiu* 国外对经络问题的研究). Beijing: People's Health Press, 1984.

Wang Buxiong *et al.*, *Developmental History of Chinese Qigong* (*Zhongguo Qigong Xueshu Fazhanshi* 中国气功学术发展史). Changshan: Hunan Science and Technology Publishing House, 1989.

Zhu Lian, *New Acupuncture and Moxibustion* (*Xin Zhenjiu Xue* 新针灸学). Beijing: People's Press, 1951.

References in English

Cheng Xinnong *et al.*, *Chinese Acupuncture and Moxibustion*. Beijing: Foreign Languages Press, 1987.

Guthrie, Douglas, *A History of Medicine*. London and Edinburgh: Thomas Nelson & Sons Ltd, 1946.

Hippocrates, Vol. I–VIII, with an English translation by W. H. S. Jones *et al.* Cambridge: Loeb Classical Library, Harvard University Press, 1995. First published in 1923.

Kaptchuk, Ted J., *Chinese Medicine – The Web that has no Weaver*. London: Rider, 1983.

Monte, Tom *et al.*, *World Medicine – the East West Guide to Healing Your Body*. New York: G. Putnam & Sons, 1993.

Ni Maoshing, *The Yellow Emperor's Inner Classic of Medicine – A New Translation of the Neijing Suwen with Commentary*. Boston: Shambhala Publications, 1995.

Petersen, William F., *Hippocratic Wisdom*. Springfield: Charles C. Thomas, 1946.

Index